the

BEAUTY
DIET

Looking Great Has Never Been So Delicious

LISA DRAYER, M.A., R.D.

New York   Chicago   San Francisco   Lisbon   London   Madrid   Mexico City
Milan   New Delhi   San Juan   Seoul   Singapore   Sydney   Toronto

The McGraw·Hill Companies

Library of Congress Cataloging-in-Publication Data

Drayer, Lisa.
    The beauty diet : looking great has never been so delicious / by Lisa Drayer.
        p.   cm.
    ISBN 0-07-154477-1 (alk. paper)
        1. Nutrition.   2. Beauty, Personal.   3. Women—Nutrition.   I. Title.
    RA784.D73   2009
    613.2'5—dc22   2008019442

1 2 3 4 5 6 7 8 9 10 11 12 13 14 15 16 17 18 19 20 21   FGR/FGR   0 9 8

ISBN 978-0-07-154477-1
MHID   0-07-154477-1

McGraw-Hill books are available at special quantity discounts to use as premiums and
sales promotions or for use in corporate training programs. To contact a representative,
please visit the Contact Us pages at www.mhprofessional.com.

The information contained in this book is intended to provide helpful and informative
material on the subject addressed. It is not intended to serve as a replacement for
professional medical advice. Any use of the information in this book is at the reader's
discretion. The author and publisher specifically disclaim any and all liability arising
directly or indirectly from the use or application of any information contained in this
book. A health care professional should be consulted regarding your specific situation.

This book is printed on acid-free paper.

To my wonderful husband, David, with lots of love

Contents

Acknowledgments

I would like to express my utmost appreciation to those who helped to make *The Beauty Diet* a reality.

To my agent, Stacey Glick: Thank you for encouraging me to write this book! It would not be here today without your terrific advice and insight. To my editor, John Aherne: Thank you for all of your support, especially when times got tough! I appreciate all of your efforts and enthusiasm for this book. A very special thank-you to Judith McCarthy, Julia Anderson Bauer, Joseph Berkowitz, Tom Lau, Amy Morse, Staci Shands, Heather Cooper, and the entire staff at McGraw-Hill, for your dedication to this project.

I am extremely grateful to Melissa Gaman, the most talented chef ever! Thank you for your hard work, diligence, and creativity in developing the most delicious Beauty Diet recipes, incorporating the Top 10 Beauty Foods. You are a dream to work with. To Nellie Sabin: I am convinced you work miracles! I am forever grateful for all of the hard work you put into this book. Thank you for all of your time and effort in making the manuscript the best it can be. To my fabulous dietetic intern, Anar Allidina: Thank you for all of your supporting research on the Top 10 Beauty Foods and "Beauty Myths."

A very special thank-you to Julie May, for your wonderful insight and hard work in helping to bring *The Beauty Diet* full circle, and to the amazing beauty publicist Madeline Johnson, for your great enthusiasm in spreading the word about *The Beauty Diet* wherever you go!

My deepest appreciation and thanks to my wonderful family, for their love, support, and encouragement: my extraordinary parents, Barbara and Barry Drayer, who—with their love, patience, and guidance—made me who I am today; my very special brother, Jeff, who is near and dear to my heart; my loving grandparents, Edie and Bernie Cooper and Sylvia and Nat Drayer, who mean the world to me; and my wonderful new parents, Dolores and Edwin Strumeyer, whom I am so lucky to have in my life.

Last but not least, a big hug and kiss to my loving husband, David: Thank you for all of your support and guidance during every stage of this book, and for showing me firsthand the meaning of beauty from the inside out. I am so lucky to have you as my partner in life, and I cannot imagine this road without you. I love you.

Introduction

As a beauty nutritionist, helping people look and feel their best is what I do for a living. Most of my clients are women for whom looking great is a high priority. And I mean *high priority*! Whether it's a bride-to-be who wants glowing skin on her big day, a television anchor who needs to appear polished in front of the cameras, or a model whose business is her looks, my clients must look terrific. I advise all kinds of people, from New York moms who maintain a high standard of attractiveness for their active lifestyle to those in business and politics who need to look stunning for their events and media coverage. Behind closed doors, I help my clients lose weight, counteract years of sun exposure, and resist the effects of aging—not with drastic surgery or expensive potions, but with everyday foods you can find at your supermarket.

Any woman would like to have a trim figure, glowing skin, glossy hair, shapely fingernails, bright eyes, and a captivating smile. Happily *The Beauty Diet* makes all these possible—*plus* it gives you the high energy and mental clarity that come from nourishing your body and brain with nutrient-rich foods.

As a woman in my 30s, I am concerned about keeping a youthful appearance more than ever before. The many advertisements for beauty-related products and procedures tell me I'm not alone. I am in the company of many friends, clients, and colleagues who are looking for ways to prevent the signs of aging and enhance their beauty. Women are staying active and beautiful longer than ever before, and I am excited to share my expert advice about eating for beauty with women from all walks of life.

How did I get started with beauty nutrition? I love reading studies and articles that reveal new facts and offer sound antiaging advice. In fact, I am a pack rat when it comes to this kind of information. If you open my file cabinet, you'll find dozens of pink file folders, all labeled according to topic. My "skin" section alone includes the latest scientific research into topical antioxidants, the link between diet and acne, the effect of omega-3 fats on skin, which vitamins can help counteract sunburn, whether collagen creams really work, and more.

My personal interest in achieving wellness and beauty through diet has turned into an exciting career. I have expanded my beauty practice to include appearances on national television shows, a column in *Women's Health* magazine, and consulting work with manufacturers of health and beauty products.

So what does this mean for you? You can consider me your friend and adviser on all things related to nutrition and beauty. My goal in writing this book is to offer noninvasive solutions to women who share similar desires for maintaining their beauty, in a safe, cost-effective manner. Turn to this book whenever you are searching for answers on enhancing your natural beauty using the nutrients in the foods we eat.

In Chapter 1, you'll find important information that will help you make good food choices when it comes to staying fit and beautiful for the rest of your life. As long as you're eating, try to make every calorie count for something! Here you'll learn how to choose nutrient-dense foods that are beneficial to your health and appearance in a variety of ways. Through my experience and research, I have identified what I consider the Top 10 Beauty Foods, described in Chapter 2, which are the best sources of beauty nutrients, including proteins, healthy carbohydrates and fats, vitamins, minerals, and antioxidants. To use them in as many different delicious ways as possible, see "The Beauty Diet Meal Plan" in Chapter 9. Each breakfast, lunch, dinner, and beauty snack on the four-week meal plan contains at least one of my Top 10 Beauty Foods, so by following the plan, you can maximize your intake of beauty nutrients without any guesswork. The meal plan includes a ton of delicious recipes and, while your taste buds will be tempted, your figure won't suffer: each day averages about 1,500 calories, to help you stay slim and sexy.

I encourage you to read this book from beginning to end, because you'll pick up all kinds of useful information in every chapter. If you need information about nutrition for glowing skin right away, turn to Chapter 3. For fuller, shinier hair, see Chapter 4. For longer, stronger fingernails, consult Chapter 5. For your brightest teeth and most winning smile, see Chapter 6. For clear and sparkling eyes, see Chapter 7. And be sure to read Chapter 8 to enrich your new healthy lifestyle with antiaging, beauty-enhancing routines.

Throughout the book you'll find special in-depth descriptions of the vital vitamins and mighty minerals that help you wake up gorgeous every day. You'll also find different kinds of sidebars: each "Beauty Myth" addresses a common misconception, each "Beauty Diet Rx" offers prescriptive nutrition advice, and each "Beyond the Beauty Diet" provides up-to-the-minute beauty advice you can use in your daily life. I have also included useful information from my guest experts, which you will find in various chapters.

In the final chapter are my Beauty Diet meal plans and recipes for four weeks of spectacular breakfast, lunch, dinner, and beauty snacks—all using one or more of my Top 10 Beauty Foods. You'll be ravishing in no time!

Sound tempting? Stay with me, and I'll teach you how to make every calorie contribute to your head-to-toe transformation. You'll experience the full glory of your natural beauty and, of course, a feeling of fabulousness that you have never known before. When the compliments start to roll in, just say you're on the Beauty Diet!

Body Beautiful

I'm a firm believer in the idea that beauty starts
with a healthy lifestyle.
— *Bobbi Brown*

It's a great time to be you! Gone are the days when there was just one standard of beauty. Open a catalog or magazine and you'll see beauty of all shapes, sizes, ages, and colors. Models and movie stars are skinny and plump, tall and short, young and old. Beauty can mean ample curves or elegant angles; long, luxuriant hair or a short bob; smoky eyes or a freckled face. What's *not* in style is looking super-skinny, undernourished, and unhealthy. Today the key to attractiveness is radiant health and abundant energy.

By making the most of your natural beauty, you'll turn heads and capture hearts. If you were born with pale skin, freckles, and flaming red locks, you can be beautiful. If you have golden skin, almond eyes, and pin-straight hair, you can be beautiful. If you have ebony skin, lush features, and wild curls, you can be beautiful. Whether your hair is jet black, snow white, or anything in between, you can set your own standards of beauty because your allure is going to come from *inside*.

When you start really nourishing the beautiful body you were given, you'll find yourself reaching less often for the concealers you've been using to hide troubled skin or camouflage those dark circles under your eyes. You'll use less makeup and fewer maintenance products once your skin regains its youthful suppleness, your thick and glossy hair grows in, and your nails grow long and strong. People will comment on how fabulous you look—or, if they can't quite put their finger on your new appearance, you'll get comments like "Did you get new glasses?" or "Did you cut your hair?"

As you will read in the pages ahead, I stand firmly behind the fact that what you put into your body—including all of the food and beverages you consume on a daily basis—will come out through your physical appearance. When you eat a healthy, antiaging beauty diet, you exude confidence while looking your absolute best.

How Food Makes You Beautiful

While I have to admit genetics plays a role in how we age, it's now clear that there is a lot we can do to stay looking youthful well into our 40s, 50s, and beyond. It's good to know that eating my Top 10 Beauty Foods—and drinking my two Beauty Beverages!—can help keep our skin firm, eyes sparkling, hair glossy, nails strong, and teeth gleaming.

When I see celebrities and Hollywood legends who look especially terrific for their age, I feel inspired. So, in that spirit, here are some age-defying beautiful women. If I look half as good as they do when I reach their age, I'll be more than happy! Follow my antiaging Beauty Diet, and you may look like Raquel Welch (born in 1940), Helen Mirren and Diane Sawyer (born in 1945), Susan Lucci and Susan Saran-

BEAUTY BITE

What Is a Beauty Food?
To make the most out of every calorie, choose foods that are:

- **Nutrient dense**, meaning rich in nutrients—including high-quality proteins, healthy carbohydrates, and beneficial fats—compared to calorie content
- **High in micronutrients**, such as beauty-enhancing vitamins, minerals, antioxidants, and phytochemicals
- **Fresh**, and preferably grown locally, to preserve the natural vitamins
- **Organic**, or at least grown and prepared without preservatives, pesticides, antibiotics, artificial colors, and other additives
- **Unrefined**, unprocessed, and unbleached
- **High in fiber**, to slow digestion and promote satiety and slimness

don (born in 1946), Meryl Streep (born in 1949), Mary Hart (born in 1950), Kim Basinger (born in 1953), Oprah Winfrey and Christie Brinkley (born in 1954), Iman (born in 1955), Sela Ward (born in 1956), or Michelle Pfeiffer (born in 1958).

First, some food basics. Don't worry, this will be fun. I just want you to understand the concepts of eating for beauty so that you will make the best possible decisions for your health and appearance for the rest of your life.

When we eat poorly, it shows. Even if we maintain an ideal weight, our skin tends to break out or become wrinkled. Our hair looks dry and damaged, our fingernails may have ridges or white spots, and our teeth become stained and even cavity-ridden. Definitely not the picture of beauty! Thankfully, changing our diet is easy, and the rewards are both rapid and radiant.

What makes a Beauty Food? Look for quality proteins, wholesome carbohydrates, healthy fats, and plenty of beauty-enhancing vitamins, minerals, and antioxidants. The more healthful nutrients a food has, the more you'll want to include it in your Beauty Diet.

Protein for Youthful Skin, Strong Nails, and Glossy Hair

An important beauty nutrient, protein is the main structural component of our bodies, and it plays a key role in the health of our features. Hair, skin, fingernails, muscles, bones, organs, tissues, and cells all need a constant supply of protein for growth and repair. By nourishing our bodies with protein, we are more likely to attain beautiful hair and fingernails. Protein also is an essential component of collagen, the connective tissue that provides support for beautiful skin. To keep skin supple and slow down the signs of aging, it is important to consume an adequate amount of protein on a daily basis.

On the Beauty Diet, I recommend consuming about 25 percent of your calories as protein. Based on 1,500 calories, this is equivalent to 94 grams of protein a day. More than this amount is not necessary, and consuming excess protein (such as the amounts indicated on very low–carbohydrate diets) can stress the liver and kidneys; plus, the body converts any protein it can't use into fat. Because you do need some high-quality protein every day—it's critical to beauty!— my Beauty Diet meal plans give you the amount that you need without going overboard.

Carbohydrates for Radiant Energy

Carbohydrates provide beauty nutrients and are essential for energy, radiance, and long-term weight management. They

Protein for Beauty

Your body does not store protein, so you need to eat some every day to continuously refresh your skin cells and keep your hair and fingernails growing long and strong. Protein comes from both animal and vegetable sources, including different kinds of meat, fish and shellfish, poultry, dairy products, eggs, nuts and seeds, legumes, and (to a lesser extent) grains. Following is a list of healthy sources of protein.

PROTEIN	GRAMS OF PROTEIN
Chicken breast, 3 oz.	26 g
Lean beef, 3 oz.	23 g
Tuna, 3 oz.	20 g
Salmon, 3 oz.	19 g
Cod, 3 oz.	19 g
Shrimp, 3 oz.	18 g
Crab, 3 oz.	18 g
Cottage cheese, low-fat, ¾ cup	18 g
Lobster, 3 oz.	17 g
Mozzarella cheese sticks, 2 sticks	12 g
Yogurt (plain, nonfat), 1 cup	10 g
Oysters, 3 oz.	10 g
Tofu, ½ cup	10 g
Milk (nonfat), 8 oz.	9 g
Lentils, ½ cup	9 g
Peanut butter, 2 tablespoons	8 g
Edamame (shelled), ½ cup	8 g
Cheddar cheese (low-fat), 1 oz.	7 g
Pumpkin seeds, 1 oz.	7 g
Egg, 1	6 g
Oatmeal, 1 cup	6 g
Almonds, 1 oz.	6 g
Walnuts, 1 oz.	4 g
Whole grain cereal (Kashi Flakes) ¾ cup	4 g
Whole wheat bread, 1 slice	3.5 g
Brown rice, ¾ cup	3 g
Vegetables (frozen), 1 cup	3 g

Healthy Carbohydrates Are Rich in Beauty Nutrients

Following are some complex carbohydrates that are rich in beauty nutrients, including a variety of vitamins, minerals, antioxidants, and fiber:

- **Fruits.** Apples, apricots, avocados, bananas, berries, cantaloupe, grapefruit, kiwifruit, oranges, peaches, prunes
- **Vegetables.** Asparagus, broccoli, cabbage, cauliflower, corn, snow peas, spinach, squash, sweet potatoes, and tomatoes
- **Whole grains.** Barley, brown rice, buckwheat, bulgur, millet, oats, popcorn, quinoa, rye, spelt, sorghum, wild rice, whole grain breads and crackers
- **Legumes.** Beans, lentils, peas, soybeans (edamame)
- **Nuts and seeds.** Almonds, sunflower seeds, ground psyllium, ground flaxseed

are the primary source of fuel for our brain and muscles. The goal is not to eliminate them but to learn which ones are best and in what quantities.

Healthy carbohydrates include whole grains, fresh fruits, and fresh vegetables. These foods contain natural (not refined) sugars, plus they have fiber. Fiber-rich foods help curb your appetite, plus they slow the rate at which sugar is absorbed into the bloodstream. Low-fat milk and yogurt offer carbohydrates with a healthy dose of beauty-enhancing protein and calcium. When choosing your healthy carbohydrates, pick those that offer lots of beauty nutrients, such as sweet potatoes (for beta-carotene), yogurt (for calcium), and kiwifruit (for vitamin C), three of my Top 10 Beauty Foods. They'll provide you with long-term energy, plus all the beneficial and anti-aging nutrients you need to look fabulous.

Refined carbohydrates are highly processed, contain few nutrients, and have little fiber (if any). The natural oils, vitamins, minerals, and trace elements of the whole foods are largely eliminated during processing. Refined carbs include white flour, white table sugar, soft drinks, and commercial fruit juices. They not only add "empty calories" to your diet, they can also make you moody and stiffen your skin (see Chapter 3).

Dietary Fiber's Role in Health and Beauty

Dietary fiber is another reason to choose whole foods over processed, refined, commercially prepared items. Fiber is beneficial for your health in various ways, but what I love most about fiber is the major beauty benefit it offers: fiber keeps you slim! In fact, I often tell my beauty-focused clients that if there was a magic bullet when it comes to weight loss, it would be fiber. Fiber keeps you feeling full without contributing any calories. So, if you want to slim *down* and look fabulous in that dress, it's a good idea to *up* your fiber intake.

When you eat, say, a piece of celery, the fiber goes right through. Why? Because, unlike cows and horses, human beings cannot digest cellulose—the main substance of the cell walls in plants. Cellulose and lignin are both examples of insoluble dietary fiber, which moves bulk through the intestinal tract and helps prevent constipation. Insoluble fiber also promotes absorption of nutrients and helps get toxins out of the body in a timely manner, both of which help to keep your features in top form.

Soluble fiber (gums, mucilages, pectins) also is not digested, but it dissolves in water and creates a gel as it goes through the intestinal tract. It helps keep blood sugar levels stable by slowing digestion and also may reduce the risk of heart disease by lowering cholesterol levels.

Fats for Supple Cells

Many women I know are fat-phobic. It's true that, gram for gram, fats have more than twice the calories of protein or carbohydrates. However, you need an adequate supply

Good Sources of Beauty-Enhancing Omega-3 Fatty Acids

- **Salmon**, one of my Top 10 Beauty Foods, is an excellent source of omega-3 fatty acids. A 3-ounce serving has about 1,800 milligrams (1.8 grams). My preferred choice is wild salmon (see Chapter 2 for more on salmon).

- **Flaxseed oil** has the highest content of alpha-linolenic acid, an omega-3 essential fatty acid, of any food. A teaspoon of flaxseed oil (or a rounded tablespoon of ground flaxseeds) contains approximately 2,000 milligrams (2 grams) of healthy omega-3 fatty acids.

- **Other sources** include cold-water fish, such as mackerel, herring, sardines, anchovies, and trout; oysters; hemp seeds and hemp seed oil; walnuts and walnut oil; wheat germ and wheat germ oil; canola oil (cold-pressed and unrefined); soybeans and soybean oil; pumpkin seeds and sesame seeds; Brazil nuts, macadamia nuts, pecans, almonds, cashews, pistachio nuts, pine nuts, and peanuts; avocados; and some dark leafy green vegetables.

of healthy fats for many important reasons, including the maintenance of your beauty. Fats supply certain essential fatty acids that your body can't make but are key to soft, supple skin. These fats help to maintain the oil barrier of the skin, which keeps moisture in and germs out. Your body also needs fats to produce hormones, and fats are used as a structural component of cells. Fats in your diet allow your body to absorb fat-soluble vitamins that are key to beauty, such as vitamin A, as well as vitamins D, E, and K. In addition, "good" fats (such as monounsaturated and polyunsaturated fats) protect you against heart disease while they satiate you and stabilize your blood sugar.

Essential Fatty Acids: Eat Your Omega-3s!

The items vital to life include moisturizer, tweezers, your most comfortable pair of ballet flats, your little black book,

Vitamin C's Role in Beauty

Recommended Dietary Allowance

WOMEN	MEN
75 mg	90 mg

In addition to playing a role in the synthesis of collagen, a structural protein found in skin, teeth, and bones, the beauty benefits of vitamin C are associated with its antioxidant properties. By helping to quench free radicals, vitamin C prevents tissue irritation and damage on a cellular level, which—among other things—helps keep skin looking youthful and clear.

10 Good Whole-Food Sources of Vitamin C

1. Guava, ½ cup	188 mg
2. Kiwi, 2 medium	141 mg
3. Orange, 1 medium	78 mg
4. Red sweet pepper, sliced, ½ cup	59 mg
5. Broccoli, cooked, ½ cup	50 mg
6. Strawberries, sliced, ½ cup	49 mg
7. Cantaloupe, ¼ medium	48 mg
8. Papaya, ¼ medium	47 mg
9. Pineapple, fresh, ½ cup	37 mg
10. Spinach, cooked, 1 cup	18 mg

the locket your mother gave you, and essential fatty acids. In fact, the essential fatty acids are as important a part of your beauty regimen as the moisturizer and tweezers.

While essential fats include specific omega-6 and omega-3 fats, omega-3s are the fatty acids you need to know about. Omega-3s play a key role in keeping your skin smooth and supple. Aside from skin benefits, a great deal of research indicates that adding omega-3s to your diet, especially long-chain omega-3s from fatty fish like salmon, helps lower blood pressure, reduces the risk of cardiovascular disease, stabilizes blood sugar, enhances nerve function, and improves mood. Omega-3 fatty acids can also help alleviate the symptoms of arthritis and protect against memory loss.

How Vitamins and Minerals Make You Beautiful

It's the little things that count. Vitamins and minerals, the micronutrients in food, keep your eyes bright, your hair shiny, your nails strong, your skin glowing, and your teeth gleaming—and that's not all! Throughout this book I describe the important beauty roles that vitamins and minerals play in your body. Be sure to check out the vitamin and mineral tables, which list the best food sources of these important beauty nutrients.

Free Radicals: How They Harm Your Health and Beauty

An optimal beauty diet includes vital vitamins, mighty minerals, and generous quantities of antioxidants. These are the substances that combat free radicals, compounds that are formed from normal activities like breathing and digesting, as well as sun exposure, air pollution, radiation, toxins, food additives, pesticides, smoking, stress, excessive exercise, drugs, alcohol, and more. Free radicals cause damage—not only in our skin, where everyone can see the results, but also inside our bodies, where the damage is hidden but just as harmful.

Free radicals are no joke. The "free radical theory of aging" holds that free radicals wreak havoc on a molecular level, and over time this damage accumulates to the point where we develop problems like wrinkles, cataracts, cancer, and various other diseases and disorders of old age. The good news is that there is a way to quench free radicals and to minimize the harmful effects they cause.

Antioxidants to the Rescue

Antioxidants are substances that take hungry free radicals out of circulation by supplying them with the electrons they are seeking without doing any harm to the body. Often, the antioxidant is itself oxidized and can no longer function as an antioxidant—unless it is regenerated by another antioxidant. This is why you need a constant supply of refreshing antioxidants!

It is impossible to live a life that is completely free of all negative influences, so it's important to keep up your intake of antiaging antioxidants. Consuming these powerful beauty nutrients is one of the simplest, most natural things you can do when it comes to enhancing your health and beauty. When you eat plenty of fresh fruits and vegetables, you take in natural antioxidants such as beta-carotene and vitamin E, both of which are fat soluble and therefore help protect the fatty membranes of cells, and vitamin C, which is water soluble and helps protects cells from the inside (see vitamin A in Chapter 7 and vitamin E in Chapter 3, in addition to the preceding discussion of vitamin C). The more of these natural antioxidants you consume, the greater protection you have against the effects of aging, both health related and cosmetic.

Phenomenal Phytochemicals

Ancient cultures have known about the medicinal qualities of plants for thousands of years. Plants contain many substances that are biologically active. Some have a direct effect on the body, while others are called *biological response modifiers* because they somehow stimulate the body to help itself.

Neither vitamins nor minerals, phytochemicals are simply chemicals produced by plants, and some of them are very beneficial—especially because they have antioxidant properties. In addition to fighting free radicals, they can enhance the immune response, repair DNA damage, fight carcinogens and toxins, boost metabolism, and enhance cell-to-cell communication. Phytochemicals include polyphenols, carotenoids, flavonoids, lignans, and many more. Foods rich in phytochemicals include onions, broccoli, apples, red grapes, grape juice, strawberries, raspberries, blueberries, blackberries, cranberries, cherries, plums, olive oil, chocolate, red wine, and tea.

Beauty from the Inside Out

By now I hope you have a solid understanding of the basic nutritional aspects of food and how the nutrients in food contribute to your health and beauty. In the next chapter, you'll find all kinds of fascinating information about the rejuvenating powers my Top 10 Beauty Foods. I've done the research for you, so all you have to do is read up—and enjoy the delicious recipes that are part of your Beauty Diet! Get ready to learn how you can achieve beauty from the inside out, as I reveal to you the antiaging secrets of my Top 10 Beauty Foods. Looking great has never been so delicious!

The Top 10 Beauty Foods

Nature gives you the face you have at 20;
it is up to you to merit the face you have at 50!
　　—*Coco Chanel*

W hy do things go more smoothly when you know you look good? Is the world simply nicer to people who are nice to look at? Or is there something inside you that is making the world take notice?

When your hair has bounce and shine, your eyes are sparkling, and you greet everyone with a delighted smile, of course your day goes better. While some new Maybelline Great Lash mascara and Bobbi Brown blush may help your cause, there is more than surface beauty at work here. You are at your most radiantly beautiful when you feel good. Looking good can help you *feel* good. But feeling good *always* makes you look good!

During the day your body is busy converting food to energy. Your brain is burning through glucose, your muscles are working, your body is digesting, and free-radical damage is accumulating in your cells. At night, thankfully, your body goes into repair mode. Your digestion slows down. The levels of your stress hormones drop, and blood flow is diverted from your now-sleeping brain to the rest of your body. Your bloodstream rushes nutrients to your cells for growth and repair. Healthy fats are used to rebuild flexible cell membranes. Protein is used to grow hair, repair muscle, and rejuvenate the collagen in your skin. Calcium is used to rebuild bones. Antioxidants quench the free radicals that ravaged your cells during the day and work their antiaging magic. Mighty minerals and vital vitamins are busy refreshing, replenishing, and revitalizing.

My Top 10 Beauty Foods are packed with the powerful nutrients and micronutrients your body needs to keep your cells refreshed and in good repair. This chapter is all about giving your body the materials it needs helps keep you healthy, radiant, vibrant, and young. To have delicate, soft skin, thick, shiny hair; long, smooth fingernails; clear, bright eyes; and a brilliant, gleaming smile, you need to nourish your body from within. The more nutrient-rich foods you eat, the greater you feel and the better you look!

Foods to Fill Your Beauty Bank

Following are foods that will feed your features and enhance your appearance from the inside out. Read on as I unlock the secrets of the 10 most powerful foods for nourishing your natural beauty:

1. Wild salmon
2. Yogurt (low-fat)

3. Oysters
4. Blueberries
5. Kiwifruit
6. Sweet potatoes
7. Spinach
8. Tomatoes
9. Walnuts
10. Dark chocolate

1. Wild Salmon

Salmon (especially the wild kind) is one of the healthiest foods you can eat. What's even more exciting is that consuming the pink fish can enhance your beauty. I picked salmon for my Top 10 list because it is one of the best food sources of omega-3 fatty acids, those beneficial fats that enhance our health and appearance by fighting inflammation, keeping our cells supple, improving circulation, and helping our brains function optimally. Salmon is a beauty food because its nutrients play a key role in keeping the skin's outer layer soft and smooth. The omega-3s in salmon reduce inflammation on the cellular level that can cause redness, wrinkles, and loss of firmness.

Salmon offers multiple beauty benefits:

- **Omega-3 fatty acids.** These replenish the lipids in the skin, which helps keep skin flexible, helps reduce moisture loss, and may improve acne symptoms. Studies have found that fish oils can protect against the sun's ultraviolet rays, which can lead to free-radical damage, skin aging, and the potential for skin cancer. Other research suggests that omega-3 fats may help keep eyes healthy by protecting against dry eye syndrome. While it is possible to buy fish oil in capsules, research has suggested that fatty acids are absorbed better from whole-food sources. The beneficial fatty acids in salmon (and other fatty fish, such as herring and trout) are eicosapentaenoic acid (EPA) and docosahexaenoic acid (DHA). Technically these fatty acids aren't "essential," because the human body is capable of synthesizing them, but this process depends on many different factors. The simplest and most pleasurable way to obtain fatty acids in optimal amounts is to eat them!

- **Protein.** Salmon is one of the best sources of high-quality, easily digested protein that is low in saturated fat. To maintain healthy skin and grow healthy hair and long, strong fingernails, you need to eat protein every day. Protein also plays an essential role in the production of collagen (which gives skin its structure) and elastin (which gives skin its flexibility). Your body needs protein to make everything from neurotransmitters and antibodies to the enzymes that power chemical reactions and the hemoglobin that carries oxygen in your blood. Protein is good for suppressing appetite because it is digested slowly and does not cause an elevation in blood sugar.

- **Astaxanthin.** Salmon is the richest food source of the powerful orange pigment called *astaxanthin* (the same substance that makes cooked lobsters red). Astaxanthin is a powerful antioxidant, 10 times more potent than beta-carotene and 100 (or more!) times more powerful than vitamin E. Potent antioxidants have dynamic antiaging effects, so salmon is a food that helps keep us young.

- **DMAE.** Salmon is a rare dietary source of dimethylamino-ethanol (DMAE). This substance is a precursor to the neurotransmitter acetylcholine, a brain chemical responsible for communication between nerve cells and muscles. DMAE helps cognitive function, and as an added benefit it improves muscle tone and firmness in the face, thereby reducing wrinkles. DMAE is now being added to many topical beauty preparations, as it appears to help skin tone without any unsightly or uncomfortable side effects.

- **Vital vitamins.** Salmon contains vitamin D, B vitamins (both covered later in this chapter), and other micronutrients. Salmon is the best whole-food source of vitamin D, which is difficult to obtain from natural-food sources. Vitamin D plays a crucial role in absorbing calcium, which in turn promotes strong bones and teeth.
- **Mighty minerals.** Salmon is an excellent source of potassium, selenium (both discussed later in the chapter), and other minerals. Selenium helps the skin stay youthful by protecting it against sun exposure and helping it retain its elasticity.

Salmon is a great food choice because it tastes delicious and has all these health and beauty benefits. Salmon is generally available and affordable, and it can be prepared in myriad different ways. You may prefer salmon fillet or salmon steak, fresh salmon or canned. You may opt for your salmon raw in sushi, smoked on a bagel, broiled as a burger, baked in the oven, or thrown on the grill. There's a recipe for this beauty food to suit any occasion. If you need an idea, see my Beauty Diet recipes for Spiced Salmon with Edamame Succotash in Chapter 9.

Why Wild Salmon Is a Better Choice than Farmed Salmon

Both wild salmon and farm-raised salmon have a variety of health benefits, but my favorite choice for this versatile fish is the wild variety. The main difference between farmed salmon and wild salmon is the environment they grow up in. Wild salmon are from ocean waters and live exactly how fish are supposed to live. Farmed salmon are raised with a large number of fish in pens. They are fed pellets of ground-up fish meal and oils to make them grow quickly, and they tend to have more fat than wild salmon. Farmed salmon are given antibiotics to fight disease and dye to make their flesh pink. Research has revealed that farmed salmon have

Vitamin D's Role in Beauty

Recommended Dietary Allowance

WOMEN	MEN
200 IU (up to age 50)	200 IU (up to age 50)
400 IU (ages 51 to 70)	400 IU (ages 51 to 70)

Vitamin D is a fat-soluble vitamin that we can obtain from our diet or synthesize in our skin when we are exposed to direct sunlight. After vitamin D is consumed (or synthesized), the liver must convert it into a physiologically active form. The beauty benefits of vitamin D generally come from its ability to help us absorb and store the calcium we get from the foods we eat. This means our ability to build strong bones and beautiful teeth depends in part on vitamin D.

Twenty to 40 minutes of sunlight exposure without sunscreen, three times a week, will enable you to meet your vitamin D requirements; however, I do not recommend this approach because exposure to the sun's ultraviolet rays is damaging to your skin. When you use sunscreen, enough UV light still gets through to permit adequate vitamin D synthesis, so there is no need to risk direct exposure without protective sunscreen.

Five Good Whole-Food Sources of Vitamin D

1. Cod liver oil, 1 teaspoon	453 IU
2. Salmon, cooked, 3.5 oz.	360 IU
3. Mackerel, cooked, 3.5 oz.	345 IU
4. Sardines, canned in oil, drained, 1.75 oz.	250 IU
5. Tuna, canned in oil, 3 oz.	200 IU

Note: Milk, cereals, and breads are often fortified with vitamin D.

higher concentrations of organochlorine compounds such as PCBs, dioxins, and chlorinated pesticides—up to 10 times more contaminants than their wild counterparts. Farmed salmon from Europe has been found to have more contaminants than farmed salmon from Chile or North American farms.

Wild salmon feed themselves naturally and are not dyed pink. Wild salmon costs more in the marketplace but contains fewer amounts of manmade pollutants such as PCBs and pesticides. If you can't find fresh wild salmon, try the canned variety. It's less expensive than fresh, and usually it is Alaska wild salmon, even if the label doesn't say so. Pregnant women and nursing mothers may especially wish to reduce their contaminant exposure by selecting wild salmon over farmed.

2. Low-Fat Yogurt

I've included low-fat yogurt in my Top 10 Beauty Foods because it is a terrific source of calcium, which is especially helpful if you want strong bones, beautiful nails, good posture, and a beautiful smile. One cup of plain, low-fat yogurt supplies about 450 milligrams of calcium. That's more than the amount of calcium in a cup of fat-free milk, and it supplies close to half of your daily calcium needs (see Chapter 6 for more on calcium). The beauty benefits of yogurt are not limited to its calcium content, though. Eight ounces of yogurt has two grams of zinc, which is beneficial for your skin. Pick up a container of yogurt for its:

- **Protein.** By now you know how important it is to eat some protein every day to have beautiful hair and nails, to keep hunger from getting the best of you, and to keep every aspect of your body functioning and in good repair. Eight ounces of yogurt contains 12 grams of protein.
- **Beneficial bacteria.** Yogurt contains live microorganisms such as *L. acidophilus* that promote the growth of healthy bacteria in the intestinal tract. Lactobacteria manufacture B vitamins, help digest dairy products, and inhibit the growth of harmful bacteria in your gut. The live cultures in the yogurt produce

lactase, which breaks down the lactose. This is helpful for lactose-intolerant individuals.

- **Vital vitamins.** Yogurt contains B vitamins, which are necessary for many body functions, including cell growth and division. (Vitamin B complex is discussed in more detail later in the chapter).

- **Mighty minerals.** Yogurt contains other beauty-enhancing minerals in addition to calcium, including approximately the same amount of potassium as a banana. Yogurt can be classified as anticariogenic, meaning it fights cavities. The calcium and phosphorus in yogurt favor the remineralization of the enamel on our teeth, making our teeth sparkling and cavity-free.

Wondering what's in Pinkberry, the "reinvented" frozen yogurt? Believe it or not, live and active cultures. Frozen yogurt is a "nonstandardized food," meaning it is not subject to federal composition standards. Not all brands of frozen yogurt actually contain live cultures. The good news is that the live cultures in genuine frozen yogurt are not killed by the freezing process but go into a dormant state. When they warm up inside the body, they get back to work!

At about 150 calories per cup, plain low-fat yogurt is a slimming treat. Try to stay away from commercial brands of yogurt that have lots of fruit and sugar added. An eight-ounce fruit-flavored yogurt may contain 28 grams of sugar (equal to seven teaspoons)! Excess sugar contributes calories and can harm the natural suppleness of your skin (see Chapter 3).

I could go on about the health and beauty benefits of yogurt for several more pages, but I'll just add that yogurt can reduce your chances of having a yeast infection and may ease the symptoms of PMS. With so many health benefits, you'll want to eat yogurt "as is" or add it to recipes to give every meal a beauty boost. One of my favorite snacks is the Strawberry Raspberry Yogurt Parfait in Chapter 9.

3. Oysters

The expression "the world is your oyster" suggests that oysters have a world of benefits tucked inside their shell. These little gifts from the sea are on my Top 10 list because they are the best whole-food source of zinc (see Chapter 3 for more on zinc). People often think of oysters as an aphrodisiac, but the high zinc content of oysters is a great beauty benefit as this mineral is a major player in skin renewal and repair. It helps create collagen, which provides the structural support in skin. It also has antioxidant properties and has been shown to be a protective nutrient at the cellular level. Zinc helps maintain stronger nails, keeps the scalp and hair healthy, and helps protect eyes from vision problems. Zinc is highly concentrated in the retina, where it serves as a critical antioxidant and helps protects against eye-related diseases.

- **Mighty minerals.** In addition to its beauty benefits, zinc is essential for a healthy immune system, aids in wound healing, plays a role in our sense of smell and taste, supports normal growth and development, and is essential for DNA synthesis. Oysters are also a good source of selenium (discussed later in this chapter), which helps your skin retain its natural elasticity.
- **Protein.** Oysters are a source of protein, and we need to eat some protein every day to have healthy hair, strong fingernails, and firm skin. Our body uses protein to make neurotransmitters, antibodies, enzymes, hemoglobin, and more.
- **Vital vitamins.** Six cooked oysters have 1 microgram of vitamin B_{12} (the recommended dietary allowance is 2.4 micrograms). It is important for many reasons, including its critical role in metabolism, cell growth, and the synthesis of fatty acids (see the vitamin B complex information later in this chapter).

Selenium's Role in Beauty

Recommended Dietary Allowance

WOMEN	MEN
55 mcg	55 mcg

Selenium is a trace mineral that is not difficult to obtain from whole-food sources. Its beauty benefits are related to the fact that selenium helps antioxidants do their job. Selenium helps protect the skin from the damage caused by sun exposure, helps preserve the elasticity of our skin, and slows down the hardening of tissues caused by oxidation.

10 Good Whole-Food Sources of Selenium

1. Brazil nuts, dried, unblanched, 1 ounce (6 nuts)	839 mcg
2. Turkey, giblets, 1 cup, simmered	322 mcg
3. Canned tuna, light, drained, 3 oz.	65 mcg
4. Oysters, 3 oz.	57 mcg
5. Cod, fresh, cooked, 3 oz.	40 mcg
6. Turkey, light meat, roasted, 3 oz.	27 mcg
7. Beef, ground, lean, broiled, 3 oz.	25 mcg
8. Chicken breast, roasted, 3 oz.	24 mcg
9. Cottage cheese, low-fat, 1 cup	23 mcg
10. Egg, 1 large	16 mcg

Are you familiar with the television show "House"? In one episode, the character Dr. Gregory House is confronted by a medical mystery: a CIA operative shows signs of being poisoned. By the end of the show, House finally determines he was not poisoned by sinister counterspies but by . . . Brazil nuts!

Brazil nuts have an unusually high amount of selenium. Ordinarily this is not a problem, but if you eat lots of Brazil nuts over a period of time, you may develop selenium poisoning. Symptoms include hair loss, depigmentation of skin, and white lines across the fingernails. An excess of Brazil nuts clearly is not good for your beauty! The upper intake level for selenium is 400 micrograms per day—which can be found in less than an ounce of Brazil nuts. Stick to half-ounce portions and alternate with one of my favorite Beauty Foods, walnuts.

Most Americans do not meet their daily zinc requirements. It's easy to add this beauty mineral to your diet with flair and flavor by enjoying oysters. They can be cooked in a wide variety of ways, such as Oysters Primavera, Broiled Oysters Florentine with Mixed Greens, and Poached Oysters in Garlic, Herbs, and Broth with Mixed Greens and Whole Wheat Baguette (see Chapter 9). Of course, many people enjoy oysters best served raw on the half shell. In that case, check out Oysters on the Half Shell with Fresh Tomato Mignonette, Mixed Green Salad, and Whole Wheat Baguette (see Chapter 9). If you are pregnant, I do not recommend eating raw oysters or any other undercooked food.

4. Blueberries

With their bright flavor and unmistakable blue hue, blueberries seem to be trying to catch our attention. Today the humble blueberry is experiencing a new level of popularity, not because it has a significant amount of any one vitamin or mineral but because of its unusual antioxidant profile. Researchers at a U.S. Department of Agriculture (USDA) laboratory at Tufts University in Boston, Massachusetts, rank blueberries number one in antioxidant activity when compared to 40 common fresh fruits and vegetables. Blueberries contain many plant compounds that combine to make this sweet fruit an antioxidant superstar. I included blueberries in my Top 10 Beauty Foods because their antioxidant, antiaging, and anti-inflammatory effects protect you from premature aging. Blueberries contain:

- **Anthocyanins.** These are the blue-red pigments that also are present in red wine and other foods; they not only give blueberries their color but also enhance their antioxidant and anti-inflammatory properties. Blueberries contain at least five different anthocyanins, which boost the effects of vitamin C, neutralize free-radical damage to the collagen matrix (the basis of all body tissues, including skin), protect the neurons in the brain, and strengthen blood vessels.

- **Vital vitamins.** Blueberries offer a healthy dose of vitamin C and vitamin E. These potent vitamins have antioxidant properties, which help to fight aging by ridding our bodies of harmful chemicals that have damaging, long-term effects on our features and internal organ systems.
- **Mighty minerals.** Blueberries are a source of potassium, which helps to lower blood pressure and boost circulation throughout the body (potassium is discussed in depth later in this chapter).
- **Lutein and zeaxanthin.** These chemically similar carotenoids are important for our eyes. They appear to protect the eyes through their antioxidant effects, as well as their ability to filter out UV light. One cup of blueberries contains 118 micrograms of lutein and zeaxanthin combined.
- **Ellagic acid.** This antioxidant prevents cell damage and may be protective against cancer.
- **Fiber.** A cup of blueberries has almost 4 grams of dietary fiber. Fiber helps you feel full without adding calories to your diet, which is a big bonus when it comes to staying slim. Plus, fiber helps control cholesterol and protects against diseases of the intestinal tract.

According to the American Academy of Anti-Aging Medicine, compounds in blueberries known as oligomeric proanthocyanidins (OPCs) help support collagen and elastin. Research has also revealed that blueberries may help protect the brain from oxidative stress. Blueberries also promote urinary tract health. They contain the same compounds found in cranberries that help prevent bladder infections.

So blueberries keep you looking young, provide you with dietary fiber, and help protect you from cancer, eye problems, and age-related diseases. At 80 calories a cup, this slimming fruit has so many health benefits you'll want to be sure to add it to your diet. If you never really thought of yourself as a blueberry lover, try my tempting recipes for Whole Grain Blueberry Pancakes, Blueberry Ginger Smoothie, and Peach Blueberry Ginger Crisp (see Chapter 9).

5. Kiwifruit

Kiwifruit offers a rich nutritional reward in a small, delicious package. Inside of this small, brown, fuzzy fruit—about the size and shape of a very large egg—you'll find semitranslucent green flesh and small black seeds around a white center. Kiwifruit has a unique sweet flavor something like a combination of strawberries, pineapples, and bananas. I've included kiwifruit among the Top 10 Beauty Foods because it offers more than just a tropical touch for your fruit salad: it has an unusually abundant amount of vitamin C and other antiaging antioxidants. Kiwifruit offers beauty benefits from stimulating collagen synthesis (vital to lovely skin) to maintaining healthy bones and teeth to protecting against wrinkles and premature aging. Because kiwis are antioxidant all-stars, they can help neutralize free radicals, which otherwise can cause damage to cells that could lead to inflammation, cancer, and heart disease.

- **Vital vitamins.** One cup of peeled kiwifruit contains more vitamin C than an equivalent amount of oranges. Vitamin C in kiwifruit is integral for collagen production and the maintenance of healthy skin, and research has suggested that high vitamin C intake is associated with fewer wrinkles. Aside from collagen synthesis, the vitamin C in kiwi is essential to the formation of healthy bones, teeth, and capillaries; plus, the vitamin may keep our eyes healthy by protecting against cataracts (see the detailed information on vitamin C in Chapter 1). Vitamin C also helps protect proteins, lipids (fats), carbohydrates, and nucleic acids (DNA and RNA) from damage by free radicals.

- **Antioxidants.** One kiwi also contains 40 micrograms of the powerful antiaging antioxidant beta-carotene (see the full story on vitamin A in Chapter 7), plus it contains the fat-soluble antioxidant vitamin E, which is usually found in nuts and oils (see Chapter 3). And there's more. Kiwis are rich in phytonutrients that protect the DNA in the nucleus of human cells from free-radical damage. Researchers are not yet certain which compounds in kiwi give the fruit its extra-protective antioxidant capacity, but they are sure it is not the fruit's vitamin C or beta-carotene content.

- **Lutein and zeaxanthin.** As you read with blueberries, these phytonutrients appear to be important to eye health. One cup of peeled kiwifruit contains 216 micrograms of lutein and zeaxanthin combined.

- **Fiber.** Two kiwis contain 5 grams of fiber, which helps keep you slim by promoting a feeling of fullness without contributing calories. Fiber also helps control your cholesterol and blood sugar levels and protects against gastrointestinal disorders.

- **Mighty minerals.** Kiwifruit contains several beneficial minerals. One cup of peeled kiwifruit has 552 milligrams of potassium—slightly more than a cup of sliced bananas. Potassium is beneficial to cardiovascular health (see the information on potassium later in this chapter). Kiwis also contain magnesium, which is a major component of bones and teeth (see Chapter 6 for more on magnesium).

Kiwi is a slimming fruit. Two medium kiwis have only 92 calories. Kiwi may also boost circulation: in a study published in *Platelets*, people who ate two or three kiwis a day for 28 days reduced their platelet aggregation response—potential clot formation—by 18 percent, compared to those eating no kiwis. If the array of health- and beauty-promoting substances in kiwifruit is not enough to tempt you to try them, turn to Chapter 9 for my recipes for deliciously cool and sweet Kiwi and Melon Fruit Soup and Tropical Kiwi Fruit Salad with Vanilla Lime Syrup.

6. Sweet Potatoes

The orange color of sweet potatoes gives their secret away. Sweet potatoes are on my list of Top 10 Beauty Foods because of their big boost of beauty-enhancing beta-carotene, a fat-soluble pigment found in many orange vegetables and fruits. It is a powerful antioxidant that protects our cells by destroying the free radicals that can damage cells (including skin cells) and cause age-related disorders. The body converts beta-carotene to vitamin A (see Chapter 7), which helps keep your skin smooth, so incorporating sweet potatoes into your diet can help you achieve wrinkle-free skin. Beta-carotene also may protect skin from the damage caused by sun exposure. One cup of cubed sweet potato contains a stunning 14,260 micrograms of beta-carotene.

To help simplify the process of choosing nutritious foods, scientists at the Center for Science in the Public Interest have developed a point system. Foods are given points for dietary fiber, naturally occurring sugars and complex carbohydrates, protein, vitamins A and C, iron, and calcium. Points are deducted for fat content (especially saturated fat), sodium, cholesterol, added refined sugars, and caffeine. The higher the score, the more nutritious the food. According to this point system, the sweet potato is the number-one most nutritious vegetable! For a modest 115-calorie investment, you get a huge nutritional return.

- **Vital vitamins.** One sweet potato more than meets the recommended dietary allowance for vitamin A. When your body converts the beta-carotene from your sweet potato into vitamin A, it will help keep your skin smooth and soft. Vitamin A also is important to good vision and eye health, cell division and differentiation, normal functioning of your immune system, and healthy bones, teeth, skin, hair, and fingernails (see Chapter 7). Additionally, one cup of canned sweet potato (which weighs more than a cup of uncooked) has 63 milligrams of the wondrous water-soluble antioxidant vitamin C (see Chapter 1).

- **Mighty minerals.** Sweet potatoes help keep your bones strong and teeth sparkling with 40 milligrams of calcium per cup (more on calcium in Chapter 6). They are also a good source of magnesium (see Chapter 6), which plays a critical role in hundreds of chemical reactions in the body, as well as a source of manganese, a trace mineral that helps keep bones strong and blood glucose levels normal. Sweet potatoes also have a significant amount of potassium, which is vital for the sodium/potassium balance in the body (more on potassium a little later). I often recommend potassium-rich foods for those retaining water due to excess consumption of sodium-rich foods.

- **Fiber.** It's more exciting than you think. Fiber helps you stay slim, helps control the level of cholesterol in your blood, and helps prevent problems from developing in your intestinal tract. One cooked sweet potato contains 4 grams of dietary fiber.

If you have limited your sweet potato consumption to once a year on Thanksgiving, use my Beauty Diet to add its orange goodness to your meals every week! Sweet potatoes can be dressed up or down, roasted or mashed, even cooked fast in the microwave oven if you're in a hurry. As a fabulous alternative to fatty French fries, try my tempting Grilled Sweet Potato "Fries" (see Chapter 9).

Sweet Potato or Yam?

Although their beauty nutrients are similar, true yams and sweet potatoes are not even botanically related. Yams are large and starchy and are grown in tropical and subtropical coun-

Potassium's Role in Beauty

Adequate Intake (AI)

WOMEN	MEN
4,700 mg	4,700 mg

There is considerable evidence that a potassium-rich diet may help regulate blood pressure, maintain bone density, protect against kidney stones, and decrease the risk of stroke. Since potassium improves blood circulation, it helps to give your skin a refreshing boost of nutrients and oxygen.

10 Good Whole-Food Sources of Potassium

1. Sweet potato, 1 large baked	855 mg
2. Tomato paste, ¼ cup	664 mg
3. Beets, cooked, ½ cup	655 mg
4. Potato, 1 baked	610 mg
5. Yogurt, plain, nonfat, 8-oz. container	579 mg
6. Edamame, 1 cup	568 mg
7. Kiwifruit, 1 cup, peeled	552 mg
8. Cod, cooked, 3 oz.	439 mg
9. Banana, 1 medium	422 mg
10. Spinach, cooked, ½ cup	419 mg

tries (nearly 100 percent comes from West Africa). Real yams can be found in the United States in international markets.

Sweet potatoes have pointy ends and are widely available throughout the United States. They are so commonly mistaken for yams that you may notice the sign in the grocery store says "yams" and then, underneath, "sweet potatoes." However, sweet potatoes are sweeter than true yams and have more protein. The light variety has a thin skin and is roughly the same color on the outside as a baking potato. The dark or garnet variety has a thicker skin and is reddish brown in color on the outside and orange on the inside. If you had "candied yams" for Thanksgiving, chances are you were eating delicious sweet potatoes.

7. Spinach

Spinach is a versatile, affordable, readily available, low-calorie leafy green vegetable that is loaded with beauty-enhancing nutrients. I included it in my Top 10 Beauty Foods because of its exceptional lutein content, which keeps our eyes healthy and bright. Spinach also contains a significant amount of beta-carotene, as well as vitamin C, several B vitamins, magnesium, iron, calcium, potassium, zinc, dietary fiber, and even omega-3 fatty acids, making it a wonderfully nutrient-dense vegetable. Following are some of the beneficial micronutrients in this super-food:

- **Lutein and zeaxanthin.** One cup of cooked frozen spinach is ranked number one among vegetables by the USDA National Nutrient Database for Standard Reference (Release 20) for its content of the related antioxidants lutein and zeaxanthin. Lutein is particularly important to eye health. The human body easily absorbs lutein and deposits it in the region of the retina called the *macula* and in the lens of the eye, where lutein is able to filter light and prevent oxidation of proteins or lipids within the lens. Lutein acts like "natural sunglasses" by protecting your eyes and also helps prevent damage to your cells, keeping your skin, brain, and heart in great condition. A Harvard University study published in the *Journal of the American Medical Association* found that consuming 6 milligrams of lutein (60 grams of fresh spinach) a day was associated with a 43 percent lower risk of macular degeneration. In addition, studies indicate that people who eat leafy greens are protecting themselves against cancer, cardiovascular disease, and age-related disorders.
- **Beta-carotene.** Spinach is an excellent source of beta-carotene, a key beauty nutrient. One cup of cooked frozen spinach (boiled and drained) has 13,750 micrograms of beta-carotene, nearly as much as a baked sweet potato and more than a cup of boiled carrots!

- **Alpha-lipoic acid.** Spinach has a special gift for you: the antiaging, anti-inflammatory, antioxidant compound alpha-lipoic acid. Alpha-lipoic acid works synergistically with other antioxidants in the skin to reduce the damaging inflammatory effects of sun exposure. It replenishes other antioxidants like vitamins C and E, plus it helps regulate glucose metabolism and keep blood sugar levels stable. It protects cell and mitochondrial lipid membranes from free-radical damage and is especially protective to the mitochondria in nerve cells. This means it may play a role in preventing the effects of aging on the brain. Alpha-lipoic acid boosts cellular levels of glutathione, an antioxidant of tremendous importance in overall health and longevity and essential to the functioning of the immune system.

- **Vital vitamins.** Spinach is a helpful source of vitamin C. One cup of cooked spinach has 18 milligrams of vitamin C. Spinach is also an unusually good plant source of the fat-soluble antioxidant vitamin E, which helps protect you from accumulating damage caused by free radicals (see Chapter 3 for more on vitamin E). Previous research has suggested that vitamins C and E and beta-carotene—all found in spinach—may protect against cataracts. Spinach is also impressive as a source of folate (vitamin B_9). One cup of raw spinach has 58 micrograms—about 15 percent of your recommended dietary allowance of 400 micrograms. Among its other roles, folate is necessary for the production and maintenance of new cells, including red blood cells, because it is needed to replicate DNA.

- **Mighty minerals.** Among vegetables, spinach contains an unusually high amount of magnesium, which plays a vital role in hundreds of the body's chemical reactions (see Chapter 6). With 167 milligrams per cup, raw spinach is also a good source of heart-healthy potassium. Spinach is rich in calcium, although much of it is unavailable, because oxalic acid in spinach binds with calcium, preventing its absorption. It's also rich in iron. To increase your absorption of iron from spinach, drink a glass of orange juice or otherwise include some vitamin C with your meal.

There are so many phytonutrients in spinach that researchers have been working on producing spinach extracts—but I'd prefer it if you ate the real thing. If you like raw spinach, try my Beauty Diet recipe Greek Spinach Salad with Yogurt Dill Dressing. For something warm, try the Spring Pea and Spinach Soup with Crab. Both recipes are in Chapter 9.

The B Vitamins: The Beauty Complex

The B vitamins formerly were thought to be a single vitamin, but further research showed that they are distinct vitamins that often coexist in the same foods. Generally the term *B vitamins* refers to the eight different types of vitamin B that, taken together, are called the *vitamin B complex*.

The B vitamins work together and are interdependent. Some B vitamins require other B vitamins for synthesis or activation. Together the vitamin B complex is needed to promote cell growth and division and maintain metabolism and muscle tone, as well as healthy skin, hair, and eyes:

- **B_1 (thiamine)** plays an important role in helping the body metabolize carbohydrates to produce energy. It is essential to normal growth and development and helps maintain the proper functioning of the heart and the nervous and digestive systems. Foods naturally high in thiamine include spinach, peas, liver, beef, pork, legumes, bananas, and whole grains. The RDA for women is 1.1 mg; for men, 1.2 mg.
- **B_2 (riboflavin)** is used in a wide variety of cellular processes and helps metabolize fats, carbohydrates, and proteins. Foods naturally high in riboflavin include milk, cheese, meat, liver, fish, yogurt, eggs, soybeans, and bananas. Exposure to

light destroys riboflavin. The RDA for women is 1.1 mg; for men, 1.3 mg.

- **B$_3$ (niacin)** is needed for energy production in cells and helps with DNA repair. It also helps remove toxins from the body. Supplemental niacin can cause facial flushing. Foods naturally high in niacin include organ meats, chicken, salmon, tuna, nuts, legumes, and many fruits and vegetables. The RDA for women is 14 mg per day; for men, 16 mg.

- **B$_5$ (pantothenic acid)** is critical to the metabolism of carbohydrates, fats, and proteins. Foods naturally high in pantothenic acid include eggs, whole grain cereals, legumes, and meat, although it is found in some quantity in nearly every food. The Adequate Intake (AI) for women and men is 5 mg.

- **B$_6$ (pyridoxine)** plays a role in the functioning of over 100 enzymes, including those that synthesize neurotransmitters. It helps the body metabolize proteins and carbohydrates and helps maintain red blood cells. Pyridoxine plays a role in the all-important balancing of sodium and potassium (potassium is discussed more fully earlier in this chapter). Foods naturally high in pyridoxine include salmon, chicken, turkey, bananas, spinach, and potatoes. The RDA for women and men up to age 50 is 1.3 mg; for women 51 and up, 1.5 mg; for men 51 and up, 1.7 mg.

- **B$_7$ (biotin)** is sometimes called "the beauty vitamin" because it is important for healthy skin and hair. Biotin helps produce energy during aerobic respiration, helps synthesize fatty acids, and plays a role in metabolizing protein. Usually the "friendly" bacteria in the intestinal tract make enough biotin to meet the body's needs. The Adequate Intake (AI) for women and men is 30 micrograms.

- **B$_9$ (folate)** plays an important role in many body processes. Folate is widely available; rich sources include leafy vegetables, dried legumes, fruits and vegetables, whole grains, meat and poultry. Folic acid is the synthetic form of the vitamin that is used in supplements and fortified foods. Folate helps with many jobs in the body, including cell maintenance and repair, DNA synthesis, and the formation of red and white blood cells. The RDA for women and men is 400 micrograms, but women who are pregnant or planning to become pregnant should consume 600 micrograms a day because folic acid protects against neural tube defects in the baby.

- **B$_{12}$ (cobalamin or cyanocobalamin)** plays a role in growth and development, helps brain function, and contributes to the formation of red blood cells. It is involved in the metabolism of every cell of the body, affecting not only DNA synthesis but also the synthesis of fatty acids and energy production. B$_{12}$ can be found naturally only in animal sources, such as clams, salmon, oysters, beef, chicken, turkey, milk, and cheese. The RDA for women and men is 2.4 micrograms.

8. Tomatoes

I added tomatoes to my list of Top 10 Beauty Foods because they provide the greatest amount of the antiaging antioxidant lycopene, the bright red carotenoid pigment that gives tomatoes, watermelons, and pink grapefruit their distinctive color. Believe it or not, tomatoes are one food I encourage you to enjoy processed. The lycopene in tomatoes is actually more easily absorbed by the body after it is processed into juice, sauce, ketchup, or canned tomato puree. Ounce for ounce, the greatest source is canned tomato paste. It's a great staple to keep in your pantry to add to soups or stews for an antioxidant boost.

- **Lycopene.** This powerful antiaging antioxidant is thought to have the highest antioxidant activity of all the carotenoids. Because of its antioxidant effects, lycopene may help protect against cardiovascular disease, cancer, macular degeneration, and possibly other diseases, such as diabetes and osteoporosis. One study that involved eating 16 milligrams of tomato paste every day for several weeks showed that ingesting lycopene may protect against sunburn.

- **Additional antioxidants.** Tomatoes contain other antioxidants that work hard to protect you from internal damage, including beta-carotene (see the vitamin A information in Chapter 7), vitamin C (see Chapter 1), and vitamin E (see Chapter 3). These antioxidants are known for their anti-inflammatory and antiaging properties. In addition, tomatoes contain the related antioxidants lutein and zeaxanthin, which are important to eye health.

- **Mighty minerals.** Tomatoes contain calcium, which you need for strong bones and teeth (see Chapter 6); iron, which benefits both your hair and your red blood cells (see Chapter 4); magnesium, which plays a role in over 300 chemical reactions in the body (see Chapter 6); and potassium, which helps regulate blood pressure and improves blood circulation (see the information in this chapter). Good blood circulation means efficient delivery of oxygen and nutrients to cells, ultimately giving you a healthy, radiant glow.

It seems like nature decided to put a powerful combination of antiaging antioxidants into the beautiful and tasty package we call the tomato. You'll think of a hundred ways to add tomatoes to your diet, from putting a thick, vine-ripened slice on your veggie burger to adding canned tomatoes to your favorite chili recipe. I highly recommend the Fire-Roasted Tomato Soup in Chapter 9.

9. Walnuts

Smooth skin tone, healthy hair, vibrant eyes, and strong bones can all be attributed to the dominant nutrients found in walnuts. I've included walnuts among my Top 10 Beauty

Foods because they are the only type of nut that contains a significant amount of beauty-enhancing omega-3 fatty acids, plus they also provide vitamin E, a fat-soluble antioxidant that helps protect cells from free-radical damage and is associated with beautiful skin (see Chapter 3). Walnuts contain:

- **Omega-3 fatty acids.** Walnuts contain alpha-linolenic acid, an essential omega-3 fatty acid. In addition to their beauty benefits, including keeping skin smooth and supple, omega-3s have been shown to protect against high blood pressure and heart disease, promote better cognitive function, and contribute to bone strength. They also have anti-inflammatory benefits that help relieve the symptoms of inflammatory skin diseases such as eczema and psoriasis, as well as asthma and rheumatoid arthritis. According to the Institute of Medicine, the recommended intake for alpha-linolenic acid is 1.1 grams per day (slightly more for men and pregnant women). One-quarter of a cup of dried walnut halves (about 12) contains 2.27 grams of alpha-linolenic acid, making walnuts an easy way to get our omega-3s.
- **Vitamin E.** This important antioxidant helps protect cells from free radicals that cause aging. Vitamin E is also an important nutrient for healthy, smooth skin. It helps to boost our immune system and may also keep our eyes bright by reducing the risk of cataracts.
- **L-arginine.** Walnuts contain relatively high levels of the essential amino acid L-arginine, which plays a special role in the body because it is converted into nitric oxide—a chemical that allows blood vessels to relax, bringing oxygen and nutrients to your cells and promoting good circulation to your skin. Nitric oxide also acts as a neurotransmitter in the brain and helps the immune system function. L-arginine is of particular interest to people with hypertension, so walnuts can serve as a great addition to their diets.

- **Mighty minerals.** Walnuts contain both manganese and copper. Both minerals help enzymes that are important in antioxidant defenses. Copper contributes to hair color, and a deficiency of copper can cause changes in the pigment of hair.
- **Ellagic acid.** This antiaging antioxidant compound supports the immune system and appears to have cancer-fighting properties. Ellagic acid not only helps protect healthy cells from free-radical damage but also helps break down toxins and helps prevent cancer cells from reproducing.
- **Melatonin.** This hormone is more familiar for regulating sleep—remember to get your beauty rest!—but it also is a powerful antioxidant, so it gives your skin a beauty boost.

A comprehensive study published in the *American Journal of Clinical Nutrition* ranked the antioxidant content of different foods, and walnuts are among the top items. When nuts and seeds are ranked according to their antioxidant content, walnuts come in first (followed by pecans).

Many people are cautious about eating nuts, but research supports eating a small number of walnuts throughout your day. In fact, research has revealed that eating just four walnuts a day for three weeks significantly increases blood levels not only of alpha-linolenic acid, the essential omega-3 fatty acid, but also of its longer chain derivative, eicosapentaenoic acid. Additionally, several studies have demonstrated that walnuts are a heart-healthy food. In fact, the U.S. Food and Drug Administration (FDA) recently approved a qualified health claim describing the heart-protective effects of walnuts.

Walnuts are a fantastic way to add nutrients, taste, and crunch to your diet. You can eat them by themselves or throw a handful into your cereal, salad, or stir-fry. You'll be happy to eat them when you try my delicious recipes for Spiced Walnuts and Oven-Crunchy Walnut Chicken Tenders (see Chapter 9).

10. Dark Chocolate

Chocolate may be described as "sinfully delicious," but in fact it is a heavenly food with many virtues. I've included dark chocolate on my list of Top 10 Beauty Foods because it is a treat for your skin as well as your taste buds. Scientific articles published in the *Journal of the American Medical Association* and other journals reveal that dark chocolate contains as many polyphenols as red wine and has potent antioxidant, antiaging properties. Dark chocolate contains many natural chemicals, including the beneficial flavonoids epicatechin and gallic acid, which are plant compounds that possess antioxidant properties. If you've been reading this book from the beginning, you know that antioxidants rid the body of free radicals, prevent the cell damage caused by free radicals, and help protect your appearance from the signs of aging.

Talk about beauty benefits from this delicious treat: a study that involved drinking cocoa (imagine!) showed an increase in blood flow to skin tissue, with improved skin hydration and reduced roughness and scaling among the female study participants. Dark chocolate also appears to protect skin against the damage caused by sun exposure, keeping the skin moist, smooth, and less scaly (see Chapter 3). Topical chocolate skin products are currently available, and chocolate-based treatments have become increasingly popular at spas throughout the country.

Godiva, Neuhaus, Ghirardelli—these decadent dark chocolate treats should be savored on any day, not just on special occasions! While chocolate lovers would argue that any chocolate is delicious, not all chocolates are created equal, and the health effects of chocolate depend on how it is processed. "Dutch processed" cocoa has far fewer health benefits than raw cocoa powder, and the health benefits of eating chocolate are negated in milk chocolate. The proteins in milk bind to the antioxidants and make them less bioavailable. Another reason to avoid commercial milk chocolate: according to the FDA, it may contain as little as 10 percent actual chocolate. The rest can be made up of cocoa butter, milk, sweeteners, natural or artificial flavors, and emulsifiers.

When it comes to the health benefits of your favorite kind of chocolate, the most important factor is whether the natural flavanols have been retained in the final product. Typically, the darker the chocolate, the better it is for you, since dark chocolate has the most antioxidants. The percentage of cacao in a product—often given on the label—gives you an idea of the richness of the chocolate taste, but it does not always reflect the flavanol content. Seeing "60% cacao" or "70% cacao" on the label does not guarantee that the product has higher levels of flavanols. This is because manufacturers sometimes remove the flavanols because of their bitter taste. An article in the British medical journal *Lancet* notes that cocoa solids can be darkened even as the natural flavanols are removed, producing a dark chocolate with fat, sugar, and calories but no health benefits.

Some manufacturers have gone to extra efforts to retain more flavanols in their chocolate as a selling point. The Mars company makes two products high in flavanols, Dove dark chocolate and CocoaVia, as well as Cocoapro cocoa powder. The more processes the chocolate is put through (such as fermentation, alkalizing, roasting), the more flavanols are lost.

You probably don't need extra encouragement to eat chocolate, but if you're looking for a special treat, try my recipe for Dark Chocolate–Dipped Frozen Bananas (see Chapter 9).

TIPS FOR SELECTING CHOCOLATE

1. For the greatest nutritional boost, choose dark chocolate. Milk chocolate and white chocolate may be delicious, but they do not have any health or beauty benefits. In general, flavanol content in chocolate products, from highest to lowest, goes like this:

BEAUTY MYTH

Chocolate Causes Acne

Last Valentine's Day my friend told me she was watching Jay Leno on television when he made a joke about the chocolate in Valentine's candy giving your sweetheart acne. I wanted to set him straight and tell him, "No, Jay! Somebody gave you the wrong information. That's a myth!" Of course, the correct information would have spoiled the joke.

Contrary to popular belief, acne is not caused by chocolate. So what exactly does cause our unwanted blemishes? For one, hormonal shifts may be to blame. Changing hormone levels in women can result in acne two to seven days before your menstrual period starts. Other skin-challenging factors include stress, pollution, and high humidity. Interestingly, some recent research has suggested that lots of highly refined carbohydrates may contribute to acne (more on this in Chapter 3). So, do what you can to minimize these pimple producers—but keep the dark chocolate on hand! The flavanols in cocoa have been shown to improve skin structure and blood flow, making small amounts of dark chocolate a legitimate, and delectable, part of your skin-care regimen. Just be sure to limit your portion sizes.

- Natural cocoa powder
- Unsweetened baking chocolate
- Dark chocolate
- Semisweet chocolate baking chips
- Milk chocolate

2. Choose natural cocoa over "Dutch processed" cocoa, which has been treated with an alkali to give it a milder flavor. This process strips the cocoa of its natural flavanols.

3. Buy chocolate that is at least 60 percent cacao. As just mentioned, it won't necessarily mean the product is high in flavanols since some manufacturers remove them to eliminate their bitter taste, but it's a better bet than chocolate with lower percentages.

4. Keep portions small to avoid excess calories. One ounce of dark chocolate contains about 150 calories. If you overindulge, the sugar and fat content of the chocolate will negate any benefits from the antioxidants!

Beauty Beverage: Water

Every system in the body depends on water. About 70 percent of our body weight is water. Our blood is about 85 percent water. Our muscles are about 75 percent water. Even 20 percent of our bones is water. This helps explain why we can live for weeks without food, but only days without water.

Drinking enough water keeps us hydrated from the inside out and helps keep our skin healthy, soft, smooth, and glowing. Water plays a key role in maintaining skin's elasticity and suppleness. It is the cheapest moisturizer around. I find that when my skin is hydrated, wrinkles are less noticeable, and my skin looks more plump.

Our kidneys and liver work hard to get rid of toxins in our bodies, and they depend on water to do their job. Additionally, water regulates our body temperature, keeps our joints lubricated, helps prevent infections, and carries nutrients to our cells.

Drinking water keeps you slim, and if you are looking to lose weight, water can help you shed pounds. Water has zero calories, so choose it over soda or juice. Drink it before each meal and it will curb your appetite and make you feel full. Interestingly, research has revealed that water-rich foods like salads, vegetables, and soups can also help you lose weight. Consuming these foods before you eat helps you consume fewer calories overall during a meal.

Bottled or filtered water is cleaner and therefore better for our bodies. The filtration process eliminates contaminants such as pollutants, parasites that cause illness (*Cryp-*

tosporidium and *Giardia*), and toxic metals such as lead and mercury. I also recommend drinking filtered water because of the taste. Filters can reduce chlorine and remove bad taste or odors, so your water is much more refreshing and palatable.

The Institute of Medicine (part of the National Academy of Sciences) recommends that women aim for 11 8-ounce cups of fluids, and men for 15½ cups—but this includes all beverages and water-rich foods, like fruits, vegetables, and soups. In general, one quart of water is needed daily for every 50 pounds of body weight.

Most people can use their thirst as a guide, except for older adults and those who exercise, because the thirst mechanism doesn't work optimally for these two groups. As you age, your sense of thirst diminishes. Also, when you exercise intensely, you can lose fluids so quickly that your brain doesn't have enough time to alert you to drink more. In that case, drink even when you're not necessarily thirsty.

To help you get your quota of water each day:

- Drink a glass of water as soon as you get up.
- Every morning, fill a 64-ounce (or larger) container with water for the day. When you drink all the water in the container, you have met your daily water requirement.
- Drink water before and after meals and snacks.
- Add slices of lemon, lime, or orange to water for a hint of flavor.
- Eat more soup.
- Enjoy water breaks instead of coffee or tea breaks.
- Take a water bottle with you to work and when running errands. Definitely remember to bring water when you're taking an airplane flight, as the air in the cabin is drying.
- Keep a mug of water on your desk to sip as you work at the computer.
- Whenever you pass a water fountain, stop and take a drink.

- At social gatherings, substitute sparkling water for alcoholic drinks, alternate them, or choose drinks that include water, club soda, or tonic.

Water is the number-one calorie-free drink that does wonders for your health. It purifies your system and keeps the cells in your body filled with nutrients. Water not only helps your internal organs perform at its best—safeguarding you from many diseases—but also works externally by providing moisture to your skin and ensuring a bright and radiant glow.

Beauty Beverage: Green Tea

Green tea is a multipurpose drink that is a great substitute for coffee, giving you a caffeine kick while at the same time offering you a generous dose of powerful beauty agents. This calorie-free and antioxidant-rich wonder drink helps protect your skin from the dangerous effects of the sun, giving you a wrinkle-free, smooth complexion.

Green tea is the only tea that contains a significant amount of the antioxidant epigallocatechin gallate (EGCG). (Both green and black tea have about eight times the polyphenols found in fruits and vegetables, but green tea, unlike black and oolong tea, is not fermented, so the active ingredients remain unaltered.) This wonder nutrient hunts for cell-damaging free radicals in the body and detoxifies them. The potential health benefits of EGCG include improved cardiovascular health, enhanced weight loss, and protection from the damage caused by ultraviolet light. Increased consumption of green tea has been shown to reduce the risk of skin, breast, lung, colon, esophageal, and bladder cancers.

While I recommend consuming green tea for its health and beauty benefits, green tea can be applied topically too. One recent study from the University of Alabama notes that

BEAUTY BITE

The "Dirty Dozen"

All produce offers nutrients that can enhance beauty, but unfortunately some fruits and vegetables are particularly susceptible to contamination from pesticides, making them less desirable than others. The following list was compiled by the nonprofit Environmental Working Group, a Washington-based lobbying and advocacy organization, and was based on nearly 43,000 tests for pesticides on produce collected by the U.S. Department of Agriculture and the U.S. Food and Drug Administration between 2000 and 2004. These fruits and vegetables have thin skins that make it easier for pesticides to penetrate. Pregnant women and children under two should choose organic versions of these foods when available.

1. Peaches (highest pesticide load)
2. Apples
3. Sweet bell peppers
4. Celery
5. Nectarines
6. Strawberries
7. Cherries
8. Lettuce
9. Imported grapes
10. Pears
11. Spinach
12. Potatoes

topical treatment of green tea polyphenols and EGCG *or* oral consumption of green tea polyphenols resulted in prevention of UVB-induced inflammatory responses, immunosuppression and oxidative stress, the biomarkers of several skin

The good news is that some produce is consistently cleaner—the clean dozen! The thicker skins on this group of produce are tough for pesticides to penetrate.

1. Onions (lowest pesticide load)

2. Avocados

3. Sweet corn (frozen)

4. Pineapples

5. Mangoes

6. Sweet peas (frozen)

7. Asparagus

8. Kiwi

9. Bananas

10. Cabbage

11. Broccoli

12. Eggplant

Organic strawberries and corn appear to have higher levels of antioxidants than their conventional counterparts, according to a recent study. Another study found that organic produce has higher levels of vitamins and minerals—specifically vitamin C, iron, magnesium, and phosphorus. More studies need to be performed, however, before definitive conclusions on the nutritional status of organically grown foods can be drawn.

diseases. This article points out that green tea polyphenols are photoprotective in nature and that green tea may help prevent solar UVB light–induced skin disorders, including photoaging, melanoma, and nonmelanoma skin cancers. In another recent study by Jennifer Gan-Wong, M.D., a topical green tea cream was tested against a 4 percent benzoyl peroxide solution on people with moderate to severe acne. The results from the study revealed that green tea was just as effective in treating acne as the benzoyl peroxide.

Last, green tea may help keep you slim. In a weight-loss study published in the *American Journal of Clinical Nutrition*, researchers looked at the effects of green tea catechins on body fat reduction and weight loss. Study participants were divided into two groups. For three months, the first group drank a bottle of oolong tea fortified with green tea extract containing 690 milligrams of catechins, and the other group drank a bottle of oolong tea with 22 milligrams of catechins. Other elements in their diets were kept constant. After three months, the study showed that those who drank the green tea extract lost more weight (5.3 pounds vs. 2.9 pounds) and experienced a significantly greater decrease in body mass index (BMI), waist size, and total body fat. Also, low-density lipoprotein (LDL) cholesterol went down in the participants who drank the green tea extract. Researchers concluded that catechins in green tea not only help burn calories and lower LDL cholesterol but may also help reduce body fat.

Now get ready to learn about feeding your features for more beautiful skin, hair, nails, teeth, and eyes.

Nutrition for Smooth, Glowing, Clear, Taut Skin

3

Though we travel the world over to find the beautiful, we must carry it with us or we find it not.
—*Ralph Waldo Emerson*

Since beauty is my business, I'm always on the lookout for the latest trends in fashion and cosmetics. There are worse jobs than reading glossy magazines and noting Hollywood trends to see what's new! I love watching the Oscars with my friends, since they all have completely different tastes and opinions and their discussions get very lively. But while everyone else is critiquing the gowns and shoes and jewelry, I am looking at the stars' flawless skin and expert makeup. These are people who *really* know how to look good.

Their interest in beauty isn't just personal, it's professional. A great dress may get them attention on the red carpet, but a gorgeous complexion will get them the close-up when the cameras are rolling.

Do you have to be a celebrity to have movie star skin? Absolutely not! Gwyneth Paltrow may get exfoliating facial scrubs made with diamonds, but I can tell you how to boost the circulation to your skin by eating the right radiance-inducing foods. Scarlett Johansson was rumored to have *three* people carrying umbrellas to shield her from the sun, but I can show you how to protect your skin with an antioxidant-rich diet. The best beauty secret isn't a secret at all: when you eat well, you create star-quality skin from the inside out.

You Were Born with Beautiful Skin

Once upon a time you had plump little cheeks and super-soft skin that lifted effortlessly into your baby smiles. When you woke up from a nap, your skin would be glowing and moist and irresistibly kissable. Come on, it wasn't that long ago!

Being skin is hard work, so over the years your skin has lost some of the suppleness it used to have. As the largest organ in the body, your skin has been busy regulating your body temperature and maintaining a barrier between you and the environment. It has been assaulted by soaps and sunlight and buffeted by dry winds. It has protected your organs from ultraviolet radiation, toxic chemicals, and germs. It has enabled you to sweat yet has prevented the vital water in your body from evaporating. It has given your face beautiful expressions, made you blush, and allowed you to feel soft caresses. Your skin has endowed you with your distinctive hair and given you fingernails and toenails to polish.

Over the years your skin accumulates damage—not just on the surface but also underneath. Free radicals break down cell membranes and cause irritation on the cellular level. Your skin gets thinner, and the fat pads underneath diminish and shift, making your skin look looser while accentuating wrinkles. Collagen and elastin—proteins that provide structure and support for your skin—start to break down and are renewed at a slower rate, making your skin saggy and less elastic. With age the skin produces less oil, so it becomes more difficult for it to retain moisture and it becomes drier. The skin around the eyes usually shows the first signs of aging due to the presence of smaller and fewer oil glands there. As you get older, blood vessels in your skin become more fragile, taking away some of the radiance of youth. Some facial expressions, like scowling or squinting, start to etch lines in your face. If you smoke, drink alcohol regularly, or eat poorly, these habits will stress your skin even more. The rate at which your skin loses its firmness and elasticity depends on both factors beyond your control, such as your genetic makeup, and lifestyle factors you can control, such as your exposure to the sun, your skin-care regimen, and of course, your diet!

Your skin is a very strong indicator of your overall health. If you have not been eating a nutrient-rich diet, your skin may get oily and clogged, dry and rough, or flare up with acne. Eczema, psoriasis, and breakouts are *not* a normal and necessary part of life. Think of these symptoms as your skin trying to get your attention. They may be a sign that you are not meeting your body's nutritional needs. Once you get your diet back in order, your skin will reward you by once again becoming glowing, moist, and irresistibly kissable.

It takes three to four weeks for the skin to renew itself. Sometimes you'll want a quick fix to zap a zit and get you through the short term, but to regain your youthful glow, try my Beauty Diet and follow the super skin recommendations in this chapter for four weeks. Then reward yourself with a special event, because you'll be ready for your own close-up!

Feel the Skin You're In

I'm sure you already know what your skin looks like. Most of us look in the mirror every morning, and for some of us it's a bit of a shock. What I would like you to do now is *feel* your skin. Check the texture of your neck and face. Does it feel firm and supple or crepelike and saggy? Does it feel plump or thin? Is it smooth or bumpy? Are there places that are dry or oily? Do you feel any areas that are stiff or inflexible?

You probably think of your skin as a very thin layer, but it consists of three layers. Once you understand the processes that occur there, you'll have a better idea why it is so important to supply your skin with the nutrients it needs to renew itself.

Your Face to Face the World: The Epidermis

The epidermis is the outermost layer that protects the body from various environmental stressors. It also has cells that contain melanin, the pigment that gives skin its color. Whether you are aware of it or not, the first thing you notice about other people is probably their epidermis—and it's the first thing other people notice about *you.*

The outer layer of skin consists of dead cells that are packed into a matrix of lipids (fats). These dead cells are continuously sloughing off, while cells in the lower layer of the epidermis are continuously proliferating, at a rate of millions per day. Cells from the lower layer work their way up to the surface through a differentiation process called *keratinization.* So the dry, flat cells on the surface of your skin today were actually once upon a time thick, healthy cells from below the surface.

The most important substances in the top layer of the skin are the keratin proteins and skin lipids. The stratum corneum (topmost layer) uses fatty acids, which is why consuming quality fats will give you quality skin. It also includes

BEYOND THE BEAUTY DIET

Smoking and Your Skin

Everybody knows smoking is bad for your lungs, but it also takes a toll on your natural beauty! When you light up—or when you are near someone else who lights up—the cigarette smoke goes into your lungs, and from there into your bloodstream, and then throughout your body.

- Each lungful of smoke sends free radicals everywhere, causing oxidative stress in every part of your body. In addition, free-radical damage accumulates below the surface of your skin and ultimately leads to wrinkles.

- Cigarette smoke makes your blood vessels constrict, which impairs the blood flow to your skin. This not only makes you look gray but also prevents your body from being able to carry toxins and debris away from your tissues. In addition, it prevents nutrients from reaching the cells in your skin, so they cannot refresh and renew themselves.

- Smoking breaks down collagen and elastin in skin, which contributes to wrinkles and sagging.

- Cigarette smoke depletes your body's supply of vitamin C, which is a key ingredient for keeping skin plump and moist. Smokers need far more of the antiaging antioxidants because their bodies suffer from far more oxidative stress.

The damage smoking does to your appearance can take 10 years to appear, but it is irreversible. Smoking simply is not compatible with youthful, soft, attractive skin. You can keep smoking, or you can have beautiful skin. Your choice.

a family of lipids called *ceramides*, which have names like *alpha-hydroxy* and *omega-hydroxy acids*. Sound familiar? Some beauty products contain synthetic ceramides to replace those lost during the aging process. These natural lipids are a major component of skin structure, and they allow the skin to retain moisture.

The Award for Best Supporting Role Goes to . . . the Dermis!

The *dermis* is right under the epidermis. It is a thick, resilient layer of connective tissue that makes up about 90 percent of the skin's depth. Beneath every attractive epidermis is a robust dermis.

The dermis contains collagen and elastin, two interconnected structural proteins that create a dense mesh. Collagen gives skin its resilience and strength, while elastin gives skin its ability to stretch and snap back. Together they support the nerve endings, muscle cells, sweat glands, sebaceous (oil) glands, hair follicles, and tiny blood vessels in this layer of skin. The dermis also contains special cells called *fibroblasts* that synthesize collagen and elastin. The sebaceous glands produce sebum, which lubricates the skin and makes your hair waterproof. These natural oils keep your skin soft and supple and prevent your scalp from getting dry and flaky. When the sebaceous glands become overactive, they produce too much oil, which can lead to clogged pores, blackheads, and pimples. Later in this chapter, I'll explain how to turn troubled skin into terrific skin.

Plump It Up: The Hypodermis

The hypodermis is a subcutaneous layer that consists mostly of fat and provides both insulation and cushioning. This layer is responsible for smooth, plump-looking skin.

Seven Steps for Beautiful Skin from the Inside Out

While some factors are out of your control, you can do a lot to achieve glowing, movie star skin. When you feed your skin with my beauty foods, it will give back to you in the form of a beautiful reflection for years to come. Following are seven ways to keep your skin in top condition by nourishing it from the inside out.

1. Keep Your Skin Hydrated

Soft and supple skin depends on two things: water and fats. This may seem contradictory because the two don't mix, but your skin needs both to retain its youthful texture.

Your skin is 70 percent water, 25 percent protein, and 2 percent lipids. Water plumps up your cells and keeps your skin moist. However, keeping your skin refreshed and hydrated is a challenge because of factors both outside and inside your body. The outer layer of your skin is constantly losing water due to exposure to dry air, sunlight, chemicals, and other elements. This moisture is slow to be replaced since water has to seep up through many layers of skin cells to reach the surface. Water for your skin is even scarcer when your body is dehydrated; your body reduces the amount of moisture in your skin to conserve water for more important functions, like keeping your blood flowing smoothly. If you are chronically dehydrated, your face will look drawn and any wrinkles will become more obvious.

A little-known dietary cause of dehydration is super-high-protein diets. Water loss accounts for the rapid loss of weight at the beginning of these diets. During the first phase of a very-high-protein, low-carbohydrate diet, your body burns any glycogen that is stored in your muscles or liver—a process that releases a lot of water. Additionally, the breakdown of amino acids from protein produces urea, which requires large amounts of water to be excreted from the body. And without adequate carbohydrates, fats cannot be metabolized completely, and this leads to the formation of ketone bodies, which have a strong diuretic effect on your kidneys. Bottom line: high-protein, low-carbohydrate diets cause water loss from the body, which can ultimately affect the plumpness of your skin, leaving it dry and wrinkled.

THE BEAUTY DIET RX

For Thirsty Skin

- Remember to drink my top two beauty beverages, water and green tea, on a daily basis. Take a bottle of water with you wherever you go and enjoy green tea with an afternoon beauty snack.

- Eat quality fats to build flexible cell membranes. It is not difficult to get enough omega-6 fatty acids from your diet because they are relatively common, but you'll want to make a special effort to add more sources of omega-3s. Among my Top 10 Beauty Foods, the significant sources of omega-3 fatty acids are salmon, walnuts, and spinach. Other fatty fish rich in omega-3s include mackerel, herring, sardines, and trout.

- Sprinkle flax, hemp seeds, walnuts, or pumpkin seeds on your salads for additional omega-3s.

- Avoid very-high-protein, low-carbohydrate diets.

- If you enjoy alcohol, limit it to one beverage and drink lots of water before and after.

- Limit caffeine to 300 milligrams per day (two large cups of coffee).

So what can do you to keep your skin hydrated adequately? For one, drink plenty of water and green tea, my favorite beauty beverages. In addition to drinking plenty of fluids, it's important to consume quality fats to keep the lipids in your skin abundant and flexible. The fats you eat are incorporated into your cell membranes, helping the insides of the cells stay plumped up with water. When you don't eat enough healthy fats, skin cells become more permeable and lose moisture. When that happens, your skin may get dry and sensitive, sometimes even red and rough.

Consuming essential fatty acids helps reverse skin problems like eczema, psoriasis, and dry, red, itchy skin. Quality fats, like the omega-3 fats found in walnuts and fish oils, are a key component of the lubricating layer that keeps skin moist and supple. Numerous studies have shown that consuming increased levels of fish oils helps keep the skin flexible and helps skin retain its moisture content. In one study published in the *British Journal of Dermatology*, volunteers with psoriasis took either capsules of supplementary fish oil or identical-looking capsules of olive oil. The fish oil group had statistically significant improvement in all parameters. Another study published in the *American Academy of Dermatology* found similar results.

Finally, for maximum hydration, consider limiting your alcohol and caffeine intake. Caffeine causes water loss from your body, including your skin. Additionally, alcohol has a diuretic effect, so in excess it can dehydrate your skin. You might be familiar with the effects of alcohol on your skin when you wake up the morning after a night of drinking! Your skin might look wrinkled and dry. Alcohol can also cause redness and flushing of the face, due to its ability to dilate blood vessels.

2. Age-Proof Your Skin with Antioxidants

As you read in Chapter 1, free radicals are electrically charged molecules produced by sun exposure, air pollution, and other toxins that attack the healthy cells of your body. Free radicals damage protein, DNA, cell membranes, mitochondria, and more.

One free radical can initiate a cascade of damage. Many free radicals together can cause extensive damage. As free-radical damage accumulates, irritation develops at the cellular level. In your skin this eventually manifests itself as fine lines, wrinkles, uneven and dull skin tone, and loss of firmness.

When free radicals target skin's support structures, your skin becomes a battlefield. When free radicals attack elastin, it loses its stretch, making skin saggy. When they attack collagen, this causes cross-linking of the proteins, making skin stiff. In addition, free-radical damage activates enzymes called *metalloproteinases*, which break down collagen, leading to wrinkles and sagging.

This sounds like a whole army of problems, but the good news is you can protect yourself simply by upping your intake of antioxidants. The body makes its own antioxidants, but it can't keep up with the internal demand—especially these days, when it is exposed to toxins, pollution, x-rays, and other aspects of modern life that cause oxidative stress. Also, the levels of the body's natural antioxidants decrease with age, so adding antioxidants to your diet becomes even more important.

BETA-CAROTENE. As an antioxidant, beta-carotene protects lipid membranes from free-radical damage that can lead to skin aging. This important beauty nutrient also gets converted to vitamin A in the body, which helps to keep skin smooth. While it is beneficial and safe to consume beta-carotene from natural sources, I do not recommend beta-carotene supplements since they may pose risk for harm. Among my Top 10 Beauty Foods, you'll find significant amounts of beta-carotene in sweet potatoes, spinach, kiwi, and tomatoes. You can also add beta-carotene to your diet with foods like pumpkin, carrots, chilies, mangoes, cantaloupe, and apricots. (For more information, see the section on vitamin A in Chapter 7.)

VITAMIN C. A highly effective antioxidant and collagen-boosting nutrient, vitamin C is a multitasking vitamin you'll be reading about again for its other valuable properties. Because you can't make vitamin C, and because it is water soluble and does not hang around in the body, you need to consume fresh vitamin C in your diet every day. A study published in the *American Journal of Clinical Nutrition* is noteworthy because it examined the effect of diet, not supplements, on the skin of everyday women. This study found that a diet high in vitamin C was associated with less dryness and less noticeable wrinkles. In addition to its antioxidant properties, vitamin C promotes healing and cellular repair and is especially important for skin because it is involved in collagen production. Among my Top 10 Beauty Foods, you'll find significant amounts of vitamin C in kiwi, blueberries, sweet potatoes, spinach, and tomatoes. You can also get your daily dose of vitamin C from foods like peppers, oranges, strawberries, lemons, and broccoli (see the section on vitamin C in Chapter 1).

VITAMIN E. Since it is fat soluble, vitamin E can protect lipid membranes in the skin from free-radical damage. Vitamin E is a good team player: it works with other antioxidants to make them more effective and boosts the effectiveness of certain enzymes that are needed for good skin health, including glutathione peroxidase. Among my Top 10 Beauty Foods, vitamin E is found in blueberries, kiwifruit, spinach, tomatoes, and walnuts. Other foods rich in vitamin E include wheat germ, sunflower seeds, safflower and sunflower oils, almonds, peaches, prunes, cabbage, asparagus, and avocados. (For more information, see the section on vitamin E later in this chapter.)

SELENIUM. Like vitamin E, selenium plays well with others. It helps create antioxidant enzymes and boosts the potency of vitamin E. Selenium is important for skin because it is incorporated into proteins to make selenoproteins. It can protect skin quality and elasticity because the antioxidant properties of selenoproteins help prevent cellular damage from free radicals. Among my Top 10 Beauty Foods, you'll find significant amounts of selenium in salmon and oysters. Brazil nuts are an extraordinarily good source of selenium. Other selenium-rich foods include tuna, crab, whole wheat bread, wheat germ, garlic, eggs, and brown rice. (For more information, see details on selenium in Chapter 2.)

ZINC. This essential mineral is found in almost every cell and plays many roles in the body. Multiple studies have shown that as an antioxidant zinc helps prevent the creation of free radicals and helps guard against free-radical damage in the skin as well as elsewhere in the body. While all of our tissues contain zinc, it is especially important for skin and is five to six times more concentrated in the epidermis than in the dermis. Like vitamin E, zinc helps stabilize the lipid membranes in the skin and protects them from free-radical damage. Among my Top 10 Beauty Foods, oysters are an extraordinarily good source of zinc, and yogurt is also helpful. Other foods that contain zinc include seafood, beef, lamb, eggs, whole grains, and nuts. (For more information on zinc, see the sidebar later in this chapter.)

ANTHOCYANINS. These antioxidant phytonutrients give some fruits and vegetables their red, blue, or purple hues. Early studies suggest that anthocyanins may be particularly helpful for skin because they prevent free-radical damage to cells and neutralize the enzymes that break down connective tissue. By protecting collagen, anthocyanins help prevent wrinkles. Among my Top 10 Beauty Foods, you'll find significant amounts of anthocyanins in blueberries. Anthocyanins are also found in other types of berries, cherries, pomegranates, plums, red cabbage, grapes, and apples.

ANTIOXIDANTS ARE KEY TO ANTIAGING AND BEAUTY. My Beauty Diet is designed to provide you with several servings of beauty-boosting antioxidant-rich fruits and vegetables every day. No single vitamin pill can come close to providing the health benefits of whole, natural foods and all the nutrients they provide. In nature many different kinds of antioxidants—some identified, some not—appear together in one food. This is part of nature's plan, because antioxidants support each other in the body. Even in scientific research using supplements, antioxidants are more effective when combined.

A study published in *Skin Pharmacology and Physiology* investigated the effects of a combination of antioxidant supplements on skin. Thirty-nine volunteers with healthy skin consumed an antioxidant mix for 12 weeks. Group 1 received a combination of lycopene, lutein, beta-carotene, alpha-tocopherol (vitamin E), and selenium. Group 2 consumed a mixture of lycopene, beta-carotene, alpha-tocopherol, and selenium. Group 3 was the control group that received no antioxidants. Even though everyone started with normal skin, roughness and scaling were improved in the first two groups, while no changes were observed in the placebo group.

Since studies have reported risks with high levels of vitamin supplements, I recommend getting your antioxidants from foods first—specifically, my antioxidant-rich beauty foods and others mentioned in this book. If you find that your diet is lacking in antioxidants, I recommend taking a multivitamin/multimineral supplement, which will boost your antioxidant intake while avoiding potentially toxic levels.

THREE WAYS TO GET SKIN-PROTECTING ANTIOXIDANTS. If your appearance is suffering because you have not been eating enough antioxidant-rich foods, there are three ways to help get your skin back into shape:

1. **Eat foods every day that are full of natural antioxidants.** The antioxidants will work together to fight free radicals and will also benefit your health in many other ways. In addition, fresh, whole foods contain other micronutrients that have their own various beauty benefits.
2. **Apply topical treatments that contain antioxidants.** The combination of consuming antioxidant-rich foods and applying topical antioxidants can fully arm you with the best possible antiaging protection. Look for foods and products

THE BEAUTY DIET RX

For Boosting Skin-Protective Antioxidants
- Include lots of beta-carotene-rich foods in your diet.
- Consume fresh sources of vitamin C every day.
- Choose vitamin E–rich foods daily.
- Include selenium-rich foods in your diet.
- Consume foods rich in zinc.
- Consume anthocyanins daily.

that pack these topical antioxidants: vitamins C and E, zinc, green tea, grape seed, selenium, resveratrol (from the skin of red grapes), pomegranate, Arctic cloudberries, lycopene, quercetin (found in apples, tea, and onions), and coenzyme Q10.

3. **Take a multivitamin.** There is no substitute for eating real food with multiple, fresh micronutrients. However, if you are dietarily challenged, it's better to get vitamins from supplements than to risk antioxidant deficiency.

THE ANTIWRINKLE DIET. If you've read my first book, *Strong, Slim, and 30!*, you may be familiar with the study I'm about to describe. If not, you're about to get some great news. The study, published in the *Journal of the American College of Nutrition*, examined the diets of 453 adults living in Sweden, Greece, and Australia. After researchers adjusted for confounding factors such as age and smoking, they found that individuals who consumed higher amounts of vegetables, fish, olive oil, and legumes were less prone to skin damage and wrinkling in areas of the skin that were exposed to the sun than those who had a high intake of meat, butter, margarine, high-fat dairy, and sugary foods. In particular, processed red meat, soft drinks, and pastries were associated with extensive skin wrinkling, while foods such as yogurt (one of my Top 10 Beauty Foods), beans, green leafy vegeta-

Vitamin E's Role in Beauty

Recommended Dietary Allowance

WOMEN	MEN
15 mg (22.5 IU)	15 mg (22.5 IU)

Note: 1 mg alpha-tocopherol = 1.49 IU

Dietary vitamin E is beneficial to skin because of its antioxidant effects, which help prevent wrinkles by keeping the membranes of the cells in the skin intact. The term *vitamin E* actually refers to a family of eight antioxidants, but the one that appears to have the most nutritional significance is alpha-tocopherol, a fat-soluble version of vitamin E that is a powerful antioxidant. Topical vitamin E is frequently used in skin creams and suntan lotions.

10 Good Whole-Food Sources of Vitamin E

FOOD	MILLIGRAMS (MG) ALPHA-TOCOPHEROL PER SERVING
Wheat germ oil, 1 tablespoon	20.3
Almonds, dry-roasted, 1 oz.	7.4
Sunflower seed kernels, dry-roasted, 1 oz.	6.0
Sunflower oil, over 60% linoleic, 1 tablespoon	5.6
Safflower oil, over 70% oleic, 1 tablespoon	4.6
Hazelnuts, dry-roasted, 1 oz.	4.3
Peanut butter, smooth-style, vitamin and mineral fortified, 2 tablespoons	4.2
Peanuts, dry-roasted, 1 oz.	2.2
Corn oil (salad or vegetable oil), 1 tablespoon	1.9
Spinach, frozen, chopped, boiled, ½ cup	1.6

bles, asparagus, nuts, olives, cherries, apples, pears, melons, dried fruits, tea, and water were associated with less skin aging. In fact, diet accounted for 32 percent of the differences seen in skin wrinkling!

My Beauty Diet maximizes your intake of antiwrinkling foods, such as those mentioned in the study. Check out Chapter 9 for my meals and beauty snacks that contain these skin-friendly foods.

3. Protect Your Skin with Edible Sunscreen

I'm sorry to disappoint you sun worshipers out there, but if you want to damage your skin, sunbathe. The harmful effects of ultraviolet radiation are well established. Sun exposure generates so many free radicals that the body can't handle them all, resulting in photoaging, immunosuppression, and the possibility of skin cancer. Melanoma, a very serious form of skin cancer, is rapidly increasing: The American Cancer Society estimates that in 2008 there will be 62,480 new cases of melanoma in the United States.

Even a brief encounter between your unprotected skin and the sun can cause sunburn (medical term: *erythema*). Your skin turns red and may even swell (medical term: *edema*). Sun exposure damages the lipids in your skin and creates free radicals, which cause oxidative stress and inflammation on a cellular level. Free radicals consume collagen and elastin, the fibers that support skin structure, causing wrinkles and other signs of premature aging. Free radicals also stimulate the synthesis of melanin, which leads to darker skin pigmentation (tanning). After just one burn, the increase in cell division activity in the skin lasts for days or even weeks, making the skin thicker. With continued exposure to ultraviolet light, the skin changes in appearance and texture, eventually becoming dry and leathery, with wrinkling and sagging.

Here's an idea you can really sink your teeth into: in addition to using a really good sunscreen, you can protect the entire surface of your skin from the *inside out* by adopting an antioxidant-rich diet. To save your skin, you'll want to add a variety of photoprotective foods to your diet. Studies have shown that eating these foods reduces burning and other damage caused by sun exposure. Following are some photoprotective micronutrients that you can add to your diet. After you consume them, they are distributed into your tissues, where they provide systemic photoprotection. With a little dietary effort, and proper protection, sun damage is completely avoidable.

CAROTENOIDS. Dietary carotenoids, found in foods such as watermelon, cantaloupe, carrots, tomatoes, and mangoes, may protect you against sunburn and contribute to lifelong protection against harmful UV radiation. A recent study published in the *Journal of Nutrition* revealed that daily supplementation with carotenoids, including beta-carotene, lutein, and lycopene, helped to decrease redness in skin when skin was exposed to ultraviolet light.

- **Beta-carotene** is used to help individuals who have erythropoietic protoporphyria, a disorder that makes their skin sensitive to visible light. Sun lotions made to absorb UV light are useless to these people. However, high doses of carotenoids effectively decrease their photosensitivity by quenching free radicals. Among my Top 10 Beauty Foods, beta-carotene can be found in significant amounts in sweet potatoes, spinach, kiwifruit, and tomatoes.

- **Lycopene**, another photoprotective micronutrient, is the major carotenoid in tomatoes. Research published in *Photochemical and Photobiological Sciences* shows that photoprotective effects are evident after volunteers eat tomato-derived products rich in lycopene. After 12 weeks of lycopene intervention, their sensitivity to UV-induced sunburn was decreased. The study concluded that dietary carotenoids such as lycopene may contribute to lifelong protection against harmful UV radiation. Among my Top 10 Beauty Foods, lycopene is found in significant amounts in tomatoes.

COCOA FLAVANOLS. Many studies have investigated the effects of the flavanols in cocoa. One recent study published in *The Journal of Nutrition* looked at the effects of repetitive intakes of cocoa rich in flavanols on skin sensitivity to UV exposure,

BEYOND THE BEAUTY DIET

Protecting Your Skin from Ultraviolet Light

Following are some tips that will help you avoid aging your skin prematurely because of sun exposure. Personally, I never go outside without applying sunscreen. I love the beach, but I use sunscreen religiously and stay covered up!

- Avoid peak hours of sun radiation (10:00 A.M. to 2:00 P.M.).

- Wear photoprotective clothing, including a long-sleeved shirt and long pants. Tightly woven, dark synthetic fabrics made from nylon or polyester provide maximum protection against UV radiation, according to the American Academy of Dermatology. Tightly woven cotton blends rank second. A white cotton T-shirt won't provide much protection since it is light in color and loosely woven.

- Apply sunscreen with an SPF of at least 30 to all exposed skin—even in the shade or on cloudy days—and use it generously. Choose a sunscreen that provides broad-spectrum protection from both ultraviolet A (UVA) and ultraviolet B (UVB) rays. I prefer products that contain Mexoryl SX because the ingredient provides a high level of protection against UVA rays, including short UVA rays. Other beneficial ingredients include physical blocks, such as titanium dioxide and zinc oxide.

- Reapply your sunscreen every two hours and after swimming or sweating.

skin structure, and texture. Two groups of women consumed either a high-flavanol or low-flavanol drink. UV-induced redness and irritation were decreased significantly in the high-flavanol group, by 15 percent and 25 percent, after 6 and 12 weeks of "treatment." No change was seen in the low-flavanol group. Researchers concluded that dietary flavanols from cocoa contribute to photoprotection. (For more on the benefits of cocoa flavanols, see the information on dark chocolate in Chapter 2.)

- Wear a wide-brimmed hat.

- Wear lip balm of at least SPF 15 to protect your lips.

- Use extra caution when out in the winter, boating, or lying on the beach. Snow, water, and sand all reflect the damaging rays of the sun, which can increase your chance of sunburn.

- Stay away from tanning booths. UV light from tanning beds causes skin cancer and photoaging of the skin just like sun exposure.

- Check the UV index. Sun exposure is such an important consideration that the National Weather Service (NWS) and the U.S. Environmental Protection Agency (EPA) combined to create the UV Index. It is issued daily in selected cities across the United States to help you avoid overexposure to the sun.

- If you want to look like you've been in the sun, consider using a sunless self-tanning product that has a sunscreen combined. You might also consider airbrush tanning or spray tanning booths.

Whatever you do, don't let your skin burn. *Five or more sunburns doubles your risk of developing skin cancer.*

GREEN TEA. This beauty beverage has many benefits, but most people don't know it is an edible sunscreen. Studies suggest that the polyphenols in green tea are photoprotective and can prevent photoaging. The polyphenols in green tea inhibit sunburn, inflammation, immunosuppression, and oxidative stress due to exposure to ultraviolet light. This is true for both topical treatment and oral consumption of green tea polyphenols.

SELENIUM. In early studies, oral selenium markedly protected mice against UV damage and increased the levels of antioxidant enzymes in their skin. Selenium preserves tissue elasticity and helps protect the body from skin cancer caused by sun exposure. Selenium supplements may pose risks, however, so be sure to choose food sources of selenium. Among my Top 10 Beauty Foods, oysters and salmon contain significant amounts of selenium. Other sources of selenium include tuna, crab, whole wheat bread, wheat germ, garlic, eggs, and brown rice. (For more information on selenium, see Chapter 2.)

OMEGA-3S. Studies have shown that fish oil—which is rich in omega-3 fatty acids—has a photoprotective effect on skin. A diet rich in omega-3s raises the skin's threshold of response to ultraviolet light, so sunburn is less severe. In one study, individuals added fish oils to their diets, while the other study group received a placebo. After four weeks, researchers discovered a small increase in the MED (minimal erythema dose, or the smallest amount of UV radiation needed to cause sunburn) among individuals in the fish oil group. Researchers determined that these findings corresponded to a Sun Protection Factor (SPF) slightly greater than one. In other words, a low dose of fish oils was found to protect against the sun's rays. Other research has found similar results. Among my Top 10 Beauty Foods, you can obtain omega-3 fatty acids from salmon, spinach, and walnuts. Other sources include mackerel, herring, sardines, trout, flax, hemp seeds, pumpkin seeds, soybeans, and whole grain products. (For more information on the essential fatty acids, see Chapter 1.)

VITAMINS AND SUNSCREENS. Do vitamins in sunscreens provide additional protection against damage caused by the sun's ultraviolet rays? At least one study suggests yes: a combination of vitamins C and E in sunscreens can be beneficial.

THE BEAUTY DIET RX

For Protecting Your Skin from the Sun

- Consume more carotenoids, including beta-carotene and lycopene.
- Consume small portions of dark chocolate, rich in cocoa flavanols.
- Drink your fill of green tea, the beauty beverage with myriad benefits.
- Consume more selenium-rich foods.
- Include fish and other omega-3–rich foods in your diet each day.

The study, from Duke University, found that when pigskin was irradiated with ultraviolet light, the combination of vitamins C and E provided four times more protection against sunburn than a placebo cream. Plus, the vitamins provided protection against DNA damage in skin cells that can lead to mutations that cause skin cancer.

How do the vitamins relate to the SPF? Generally speaking, you can improve the SPF of sunscreen with the addition of vitamins C and E by a factor of 1 to 4. In other words, if you have an SPF of 15, maybe you will get an SPF of 19 with the vitamins added.

ON THE HORIZON. Would you believe the next big thing could be a topical solution that protects against sunburn . . . made from broccoli sprouts? Although it is applied topically, this substance is not a sunscreen, and it does not work by filtering out UV light and preventing its entry into the skin. Instead, it works inside the skin by boosting the production of protective enzymes that defend cells against UV damage. The topical solution can even be applied three days before you go out in the sun, because its protection lasts for several days.

THE BEAUTY DIET RX

For Boosting Circulation to Your Skin

- Consume more omega-3 fatty acids. Choose cold-water fish like salmon, mackerel, herring, sardines, trout. Add walnuts, spinach, flax, hemp seeds, pumpkin seeds, and soybeans to your diet.

- Sprinkle walnuts into your salad, throw them into a stir-fry, or put them on your oatmeal in the morning. Check out my Beauty Diet meal plan (Chapter 9) for other ideas! Other sources of L-arginine, the magic ingredient in walnuts that enhances circulation, include peanuts, almonds, sunflower seeds, hazelnuts, Brazil nuts, cashew nuts, pistachio nuts, pecans, flax seeds, tuna, shrimp, eggs, and soybeans (including edamame and tofu).

- Go ahead—drink some high-flavanol cocoa. Eating high-flavanol dark chocolate works too (be sure to check out some of my dark chocolate beauty snacks in Chapter 9).

4. Boost Circulation with Skin-Friendly Foods

Exercise brings a glow to your cheeks because of the increase in circulation, which helps keep your skin hydrated, promotes healing, brings micronutrients and oxygen to your skin cells, and whisks away dead cells and toxins. However, you can't exactly drop to the floor and do 20 crunches every time you want a healthy glow. Blushing works, but there are side effects involving your dignity. Following are skin-friendly foods that can help give you a beautiful complexion.

OMEGA-3 FATTY ACIDS. Omega-3 fats found in fish oils offer circulatory benefits by reducing blood pressure, preventing platelet clotting, and maintaining the elasticity of arterial walls. Among my Top 10 Beauty Foods, you can obtain a healthy dose of omega-3–rich fish oil from salmon. Other sources of omega-3–rich fish oils include mackerel, herring, sardines, and trout.

WALNUTS. Luckily for us, walnuts have a beneficial effect on circulation because they contain L-arginine, from which the body can create nitric oxide, which opens up blood vessels. An article published in the journal *Circulation* describes a study in which participants with high serum cholesterol levels ate two different carefully constructed diets, one that included olive oil and another that replaced 32 percent of the calories from olive oil with walnuts. Four hours after a meal containing walnuts, brachial artery reactivity was measured by ultrasound. Vasodilation improved significantly after the walnut meal, compared with the olive oil meal. This means walnuts have a direct and almost immediate effect on the blood vessels, helping them open wider to keep blood flowing freely to all areas of the body.

COCOA. A delicious way to promote circulation to your skin is to drink cocoa or eat dark chocolate with high levels of cocoa flavanols. Researchers have found that cocoa causes an increase in blood flow to the skin, with a corresponding increase in hydration and skin density. The Mars company did a study using its Cocoapro product and found that women who drank high-flavanol cocoa for 12 weeks showed significant improvements in their skin, including an increase in skin hydration and a decrease in skin roughness and scaling. Researchers attributed this improvement to an increase in blood flow to the surface of the skin. A study published in the *European Journal of Nutrition* was based on participants drinking just one serving of cocoa. Within an hour, blood flow to the skin was increased. The article noted that regular consumption of cocoa leads to a significant increase in blood flow in cutaneous (skin) and subcutaneous tissue (beneath the skin).

5. Renew Your Skin with Beauty Nutrients

Like Madonna, your skin is constantly reinventing itself. On the surface, old cells slough off and are replaced by new ones. Underneath, the cells in the dermis begin to lose their strength and flexibility. At the same time as the supporting structures of your skin begin to break down, the production of fresh collagen slows, so skin starts to wrinkle and sag. Collagen makes up 75 percent of the skin, so many people are looking for ways to restore it. It is possible to get collagen injected directly into wrinkles and to buy collagen creams that promise to rebuild the skin (they can't—the molecules of collagen are too large for the skin to absorb). The Japanese even sell marshmallows with collagen added—although there is no evidence that eating collagen will make any difference to your skin.

To rejuvenate your skin, you're going to need fresh collagen that is created on the inside. Following are some ways to enhance collagen synthesis by adding whole, natural, skin-boosting foods to your diet.

PROTEIN. Amino acids are the building blocks your body uses to make collagen, so if you want fresh new skin cells, you need to eat some high-quality protein every day. Among my Top 10 Beauty Foods, the highest amount of protein is found in salmon, yogurt, walnuts, and oysters. Other good sources of protein include fish, shellfish, turkey, chicken, beef, lamb, soybeans, eggs, nuts, and dairy products. (See the protein section in Chapter 1.)

VITAMIN C. Because vitamin C it is necessary to the production of collagen, it is important to consume lots of vitamin C–rich foods. Vitamin C has been shown to stimulate the growth of collagen when applied topically, so it is often included in all kinds of antiaging cosmetics. Among my Top 10 Beauty Foods, significant amounts of vitamin C are found in kiwi, blueberries, sweet potatoes, spinach, and tomatoes. Vitamin C is also found in foods like peppers, oranges, strawberries, lemons, and broccoli. (For more information on vitamin C, see Chapter 1.)

VITAMIN A. A key beauty nutrient, vitamin A is important to skin renewal because it is involved in the proper growth, repair, and maintenance of the skin and helps control sebum levels. We know vitamin A has special significance for the skin because a deficiency of vitamin A makes the skin dry and flaky. Vitamin A is so helpful to skin that it is used in prescription medications, both oral and topical, to combat acne and other problems. More preformed vitamin A from supplements is not necessarily better, however: if you choose a multivitamin, check that at least 20 percent comes from beta-carotene, the precursor to vitamin A. Among my Top 10 Beauty Foods, animal sources of vitamin A are oysters, yogurt, and salmon. Other sources include milk, cheddar cheese, and eggs. Among my Top 10 Beauty Foods, you'll find significant amounts of beta-carotene, the precursor to vitamin A synthesis, in sweet potatoes, spinach, kiwi, and tomatoes. You can also add beta-carotene to your diet with foods like pumpkin, carrots, chilies, mangoes, cantaloupe, and apricots. (For more information on vitamin A, see Chapter 7.)

ANTHOCYANINS. In addition to their antioxidant properties, anthocyanins help stabilize the collagen matrix by means of cross-linking. This means that as your skin renews itself, you'll want these phytonutrients available to strengthen your connective tissue. Among my Top 10 Beauty Foods, anthocyanins are found in blueberries. They are also found in other blue, red, and purple foods, including other types of berries, cherries, pomegranates, plums, red cabbage, grapes, and apples.

Zinc's Role in Beauty

Recommended Dietary Allowance

WOMEN	MEN
8 mg	11 mg

A deficiency of zinc can cause skin problems, while an abundance of zinc is beneficial to the skin in many ways. Zinc is necessary for the synthesis of collagen, and its antioxidant properties help prevent wrinkles. Zinc may also help with acne symptoms.

10 Good Whole-Food Sources of Zinc

1.	Oysters, 6, cooked	76.3 mg
2.	Beef, cooked, 3 oz.	4.8 mg
3.	Pork loin, cooked, 3 oz.	2.2 mg
4.	Yogurt, fruit, 1 cup	1.8 mg
5.	Baked beans, canned, ½ cup	1.8 mg
6.	Milk, 1 cup (any fat content)	1.8 mg
7.	Chicken, dark meat, 3 oz.	1.8 mg
8.	Cashews, 1 oz.	1.6 mg
9.	Chickpeas, ½ cup	1.3 mg
10.	Walnuts, 1 oz. (4 halves)	0.9 mg

VITAMIN B COMPLEX. The B complex includes eight vitamins important to skin renewal because they are essential to cell reproduction. A deficiency of the B vitamin riboflavin can interfere with proper collagen synthesis, and deficiencies of other Bs can cause problems from scaly skin to acne. Among my Top 10 Beauty Foods, the best source of thiamine (B_1) and biotin (B_7) is walnuts, the best source of riboflavin (B_2) and pantothenic acid (B_5) is yogurt, the best source of niacin (B_3) is wild salmon, the best source of folate (B_9) is spinach, and the best source of cobalamin (B_{12})—which is available only from animal sources—is oysters. Spinach, walnuts, and salmon are all good sources of pyridoxine (B_6).

THE BEAUTY DIET RX

For Skin Renewal

- Consume plenty of protein to build new skin.
- Consume plenty of fresh vitamin C–rich foods to help build collagen.
- Consume more vitamin A (from animal sources) and beta-carotene (from plant sources) to help grow fresh skin cells.
- Consume more anthocyanins to strengthen your connective tissue.
- Consume enough B vitamins to aid cell reproduction.
- Consume plenty of zinc to assist in cell growth.
- Make the switch from refined white flour to foods made with whole grains. You'll gain a wide variety of beauty nutrients, including silicon for healthy skin.

ZINC. Zinc is important to skin renewal because it is needed for the synthesis of collagen and elastin. Zinc has a special affinity for the skin and has been shown to speed wound healing and may improve the symptoms of acne. Among my Top 10 Beauty Foods, an amazing amount of zinc is found in oysters, and yogurt is a good source as well. You can add more zinc to your diet with seafood, beef, lamb, eggs, whole grains, and nuts. (For more information on zinc, see the sidebar.)

SILICON. The second most common element on the surface of the Earth (after oxygen), silicon is found in the human body in the highest concentrations in skin and hair. A deficiency of silicon is characterized by poor skin quality, dry hair, brittle fingernails, and arterial disease. As a component of collagen, silicon is important to the proper integrity of the skin. With age, the silicon content of the skin tends to decline more than it declines in other tissues. This has led to an interest in

BEAUTY BITE

Hidden Sugar

The sugars listed on the Nutrition Facts panel of food ingredients do not distinguish between naturally occurring sugars (like those in fruit and milk) and sugars that are added. This ingredient list will help you find the hidden sugars in food. Manufacturers use many kinds of sweeteners with many different names, so watch out for:

sugar	cane sugar
invert sugar	white sugar
brown sugar	confectioners' sugar
raw sugar	beet sugar
turbinado sugar	evaporated cane juice
honey	maple syrup
molasses	corn syrup
dextrin	maltodextrin
dextrose	corn sweeteners
fructose	corn syrup
high-fructose corn syrup	malt
rice syrup	fruit juice concentrate
apple juice concentrate	concentrated pear puree
galactose	glucose
lactose	polydextrose

"No added sugars" or "without added sugars" indicates that sugars have not been added in processing.

"Reduced sugar" and "less sugar" refer to products that contain at least 25 percent less sugar than a comparable product.

"Sugar-free" products are defined as less than 0.5 gram sugar per serving. Sugar-free products do not contain natural or added sugars but may contain sweeteners known as *sugar alcohols* that do not contribute calories or significantly affect blood sugar levels but may cause gastrointestinal symptoms because they are not completely absorbed.

If you limit your added sugar for the day to 10 percent of your total calories, and you consume 1,500 calories a day, that gives you 150 calories of added sugar to play with—the amount in one can of regular soda.

dietary silicon supplements. There also is growing interest in topical silicon-based products in the cosmetics industry. High-fiber diets contain lots of silicon, the element found in whole grains, bananas, string beans, cereals, fruit, and dairy food. Highly processed foods contain little silicon.

6. Stay Away from Sugar

We all know we should avoid sugar. It tastes great, but it adds empty calories to our diet, elevates our blood sugar levels, and throws the body into fat-storage mode. But here's another reason to stay away from sugar. Most of my clients are surprised to hear that eating sugar can sabotage your skin! Here's how it works.

When blood sugar levels are high, sugar molecules can permanently bond to proteins, including the collagen in your skin—a process known as *glycation*. This process produces chemical compounds called Advanced Glycation Endproducts (AGEs) that cross-link with adjacent strands of protein. When this occurs, the strands of protein that support your skin can no longer move freely, making tissues stiff and inflexible. This makes skin tougher, saggier, and more wrinkled. Glycation and cross-linking also can cause inflammatory responses.

You already know that cookies, soda, sugar-coated cereal, and ice cream have lots of sugar. A 12-ounce can of soda contains about 10 teaspoons of sugar. (One teaspoon of sugar has 15 calories.) The foods to watch out for are those that seem like they might be good for you but actually contain hidden sugar, such as fruit drinks, ketchup, commercially made granola bars and bran muffins, and some exotic waters and energy drinks.

7. Check for Food Allergies

Food allergies are often the culprit behind inflammations of the skin, including redness, hives, swelling, and eczema.

BEYOND THE BEAUTY DIET

Protect Your Skin's Acid Mantle

The term *acid mantle* refers to the natural covering that protects your skin, which is produced by the sweat glands and sebaceous glands. Healthy skin is a little bit acidic, which helps protect it from infection and helps prevent the growth of harmful bacteria.

When the acid mantle is disrupted, skin can become more prone to damage and infection. Many commercial skin cleansers and moisturizers have a pH of nine or higher, giving the skin a very tight, clean feel. Over time using these highly alkaline products disrupts the pH of the skin.

To help keep your skin at its natural pH level, choose topical treatments that do not interfere with its acidity. Wash your face kindly. Avoid antibacterial soaps, which tend to reduce the acidity of the skin, and know the pH of any cleansers, moisturizers, makeup or other products you use on your face. Ideally they should be slightly acidic, with a pH of approximately five to six. Having a pH outside this zone can interfere with normal skin functions, including repair and renewal.

The symptoms of food allergies and sensitivities range from mild to severe. You could have a moderate allergy to certain foods without being aware of it.

When you have an extreme food allergy, your body has a full-on inflammatory reaction for the wrong reason. It believes that molecules of wheat or egg or soy are a threat, and it wages a systemic allergic reaction that makes your throat swell up and your skin erupt in hives. Even a minuscule amount of allergen can immediately ignite another inflammatory response.

Many people have milder forms of food allergies that they don't even know about. This means on a regular basis they are eating foods that activate their immune system, causing constant, low-level inflammation.

If you know you have mild food allergies or sensitivities, don't try to get away with eating "just a little" of the food item to which you are allergic. This just keeps your immune system constantly upregulated.

If you suspect you may have food allergies but aren't sure what they are, try the elimination diet—it works! You begin by eliminating foods from your diet that tend to cause allergies. Gradually you reintroduce different foods, waiting to see if your body shows signs of sensitivity. If your skin reacts when you consume specific foods, then by eliminating any foods to which you are sensitive, you can reduce inflammation and its associated symptoms. By choosing foods that do not challenge your immune system, you restore your clear, glowing complexion.

The Antiacne Diet

Is there anything more horrifying than waking up and discovering a hideous pimple on your face? OK, I admit there are worse things in life. But when it comes to everyday problems, acne can be really discouraging.

Acne is caused by clogged pores and the inflammation of the sebaceous glands and hair follicles. When the glands in the skin produce too much sebum, the oil combines with dead skin cells, and pores become plugged. This creates blackheads and whiteheads.

There is a link between diet and acne—but it's not what most people think it is. Many of us grew up believing that chocolate and fried foods cause acne, but the real dietary culprits are sugar and foods that promote inflammation. How exactly does it happen? Loren Cordain, Ph.D., a professor of health and exercise science at Colorado State University who has studied the link between foods and acne, says that when you eat too many carbs (too often and in the wrong proportions), your body makes more insulin, which increases production of hormones known as *androgens*. High levels of androgens cause sebaceous glands in the skin to

THE BEAUTY DIET RX

For Acne

- **Avoid highly processed refined carbohydrates and sweet foods.** They create a spike in blood sugar that sets off a series of hormonal changes that cause inflammation and acne.

- **Identify any food allergies** you might have. If you have allergies or sensitivities, stay away from problem foods, which cause inflammation. Keep in mind that you also might be allergic to topical preparations you are using on your skin, including sunscreen or, ironically, beauty products.

- **Eat a high-fiber diet** that includes lots of fruits and vegetables, legumes, and whole grain breads and cereals. The nutrients in whole, natural foods are so good for your skin; plus, these foods do not promote inflammation.

- **Add omega-3 fatty acids** to your to diet help combat inflammation. Acne may be caused by taking in too little omega-3 fats in relation to omega-6 fats. Such an imbalance can cause inflammation, leading to blocked pores that cause an overproduction of oil, according to researchers.

- **Eat plenty of foods that contain beta-carotene.** The body converts beta-carotene into vitamin A, which is particularly beneficial to skin.

- **Eat plenty of foods that contain zinc.** This mineral has anti-inflammatory properties and is very effective against acne. Good sources of zinc include oysters, crab, turkey, wheat germ, tofu, and cashews and pumpkin seeds.

- **Drink lots of water** to help your body rid itself of toxins that might otherwise contribute to skin flare-ups.

Note: Drugs prescribed for acne include Accutane (isotretinoin) and Retin-A (tretinoin). These are derivatives of vitamin A and should not be taken during pregnancy or if you are planning on becoming pregnant because high doses of vitamin A can cause birth defects.

BEYOND THE BEAUTY DIET

Lifestyle Tips for Gorgeous Skin

- **Drink water, not alcohol.** Drinking alcohol contributes to aging skin by dilating small blood vessels in the skin and increasing blood flow near the skin's surface. Over time these blood vessels can become permanently damaged, creating a flushed appearance and broken vessels on the skin's surface. Drinking water keeps you adequately hydrated and your skin moist and supple.

- **Relax!** Stress and worry cause frowning, and over time the muscles in the face actually conform to that movement. Be aware of your stress level and try to relax your facial muscles during the day. A good antiaging skin-care program should include meditation, yoga, gentle exercise, or other relaxation techniques (see Chapter 8).

- **Get your beauty rest.** Lack of sleep shows up on your face as puffiness, bags, and dark circles under your eyes. Most adults need eight hours of sleep each night to feel refreshed in the morning. (If you are having trouble getting to sleep, see my tips in Chapter 8.)

secrete more oil that becomes trapped inside the pores, so skin appears shinier and pimples become plentiful. In other words, a diet focused on refined carbohydrates (those in white breads, cookies and cake, and even some salty snacks) sets off a hormonal cascade that causes excess oil production in the skin, leading to clogged pores and pimples.

In one recent randomized controlled trial published in *The American Journal of Clinical Nutrition*, individuals with acne were assigned to either a diet consisting of 25 percent protein and 45 percent low-glycemic-index carbohydrates or to a Westernized diet rich in refined, sugary carbohydrates.

BEAUTY MYTH

Vitamin E Helps Reduce Scars

Although vitamin E is the main lipid-soluble antioxidant in the skin, further research is needed to prove its effectiveness in reducing scars and stretch marks. One study looked at a randomized group of 159 burn patients who were treated with topical vitamin E for four months. After one year, scar thickness, alteration in graft size, range of motion, and appearance of the scars were recorded. No beneficial effect of vitamin E was seen in any of the patients. In another study, postsurgical patients were given two ointments labeled *A* and *B*. One of the ointments contained vitamin E, and the other didn't. Patients were instructed to apply each ointment on a separate half of their scars twice a day for four weeks. The researchers concluded that not only did the vitamin E have no beneficial effects on the scars; it actually made matters worse as some patients experienced an allergic reaction to the vitamin E. Bottom line: don't depend on vitamin E creams to reduce the appearance of scars and stretch marks.

After 12 weeks, those following the experimental diet low in refined carbohydrates experienced an improvement in their skin, as evidenced by a decrease in "total and inflammatory lesion counts." Their acne had improved significantly compared to the control group.

My Beauty Diet includes all the nutrients you need for beautiful skin and avoids problem foods with lots of sugar and poor-quality fats. By making a few modifications, you can create your own personal Antiacne Diet. Follow it closely and you should see improvements in your skin in about four weeks.

Dairy and Acne

Many people have asked me if dairy foods can cause acne. Here's the lowdown: Some researchers believe that iodine is what exacerbates acne, and dairy products are a source of iodine. In addition, farmers give their cows iodine-fortified feed and use sanitizing iodine solutions on cows' udders and milking equipment. Others believe that hormones in milk may be responsible for acne. While research has revealed that drinking milk and consuming dairy products from pregnant cows exposes us to hormones from the cows' pregnancy, the amount of hormones in the milk is minuscule compared to the amount produced in our bodies, according to Greg Miller, Ph.D., a scientist with the National Dairy Council.

The dairy and acne link has not been substantiated in clinical studies. If you suffer from regular acne flare-ups, it is most likely due to other causes.

Topical Treatments

Many of the foods discussed in this chapter can also be applied directly to your face. For example, many people use yogurt as a face mask. I have read that applying fish oil to your skin can be beneficial, but I have not tried this person-ally—I don't want my husband, David, to think I smell like a mermaid!

Many natural substances found in food are now being used in commercial cosmetics. For example, dimethylaminoetha-nol, which is found in salmon, is used topically to increase circulation. A modified version of vitamin C can be applied to the skin, and of course medications containing vitamin A are used for acne and other skin problems. I asked my friend Valerie, a skin specialist who owns the Face Studio in New York City, for her recommendations regarding food and beau-tiful skin. You can read what she has to say in the "Expert Advice" section that follows. If you are considering other top-ical treatments for your skin, be sure to check out Dr. Aron Kressel's advice in the second "Expert Advice" section.

Expert Advice: Natural Skincare Ingredients Found Inside Your Home

According to skin expert Valerie Mayo of the Face Studio in New York City, once you find the right combination of natural ingredients for your skin, you will be amazed at how radiant you look.

Following are a few suggestions from Valerie for using natural skin-care ingredients found at home to get you moving toward healthy, balanced, and radiant skin. Remember to test any ingredient on a small area of your body first, to make sure you are not allergic.

- **Honey.** Humectants attract and help to retain moisture, which is a major factor in giving the skin a hydrated and plump appearance.
- **Strawberries and egg whites.** Strawberries contain antioxidants that help the skin fight free radicals caused by stress, sun, and pollution. Egg whites have a great firming effect on skin. Mix the ingredients together and you have a winning antiaging combo.
- **Lemons.** These are excellent for lightening dark patches on the surface of the face and body. The citric acid is the ingredient that lightens the skin.
- **Oats, lemon juice, and honey.** This is an excellent combination for a moisturizing facial mask. The oats and honey hydrate and plump, while the lemon lightens.
- **Plain yogurt.** This is an excellent mask for oily and combination skin. Yogurt, oatmeal, and honey are a great combination to use for balancing the skin.
- **Milk.** Excellent for soothing irritated skin. Milk contains lactic acids, which are enzymes that help to exfoliate dry patches and make skin smooth and soft. Great for soothing mild sunburns and shaving irritations.

- **Water.** The best natural resource ever! Drinking water hydrates the skin and helps flush out toxins, which can cause all types of skin problems. Dehydration is a major cause of dry, dull, and patchy skin, as well as acne with dry patches. Water is one of the great balancers of life.

Expert Advice: Skin Treatments

According to New York City–based plastic surgeon Dr. Aron Kressel, the character of our skin will change as we age due to a combination of external and internal factors. Externally, the sun's rays and air pollutants will cause the skin to become wrinkled, rough, and darkened and to develop red spots. Internally the chronological, inevitable aging of the skin causes thinning of the skin and loss of elasticity. Following is a summary of Dr. Kressel's lowdown on popular skin treatments.

Numerous products have become available with the promise of rejuvenating the skin. What these products share is their ability to stimulate the components of the skin to develop thicker, plumper, shinier, and smoother skin. Products containing alpha-hydroxy acids are available in concentrations ranging from 5 percent to 15 percent. Alpha-hydroxy acids (glycolic acid) have been shown to improve hyperpigmentation, color, and to a lesser degree the character of wrinkles. When used in moisturizer products at a 4- to 5-percent concentration, skin smoothness has improved.

Tretinoin (Renova/Retin-A) is a prescription product that has been shown conclusively to improve wrinkles and smooth skin by stimulating collagen production. Unfortunately, when use of the product is discontinued, the skin reverts to its untreated condition. The major drawback of this product is that the skin becomes quite sensitive to sun exposure.

Glycolic acid and trichloroacetic peels have been shown to smooth skin and reduce hyperpigmentation. The higher the product's concentration, the greater the resulting effect, though with deeper chemical trauma to the skin. More peel means more posttreatment redness and crusting, which can often last for several weeks or months. Another potential complication is the development of areas of scarring or irregular skin lightening.

Treatment with laser or LED light causes a controlled thermal burn on the layers of the skin. The depth of injury depends on the type of laser and other factors varied by the laser operator. Often small variations in the settings can cause significant trauma to the skin. Just as with chemical peels, these burns can cause redness and crusting and potentially areas of irregular skin lightening. Many of the lasers/light products will require multiple treatments over several months. The hope is that, by using a less aggressive treatment more frequently, the posttreatment side effects will be minimal.

When evaluating options for skin rejuvenation, take a historical perspective. Over the years numerous products have arrived with great promise that did not stand the test of time. Clearly, if there were a perfect product, research would cease. When looking at a new product or treatment being offered, we have to look at its potential for improvement and also weigh it based on the number of treatments that will be needed, the time commitment required, and the potential for skin damage.

Nutrition for Rich, Shiny, Strong, Soft Hair

Zest is the secret of all beauty. There is no beauty that is attractive without zest.
> —*Christian Dior*

On a good hair day, anything seems possible! When your hair is lustrous and shiny, with extra bounce and body, you feel energetic, attractive, and sexy. With the right color and a terrific cut, you know you'll make a good first impression on a date, you'll turn heads walking down the street, or you'll command attention when you need it most. When and with whom you choose to let your hair down later is your business!

Beautiful, healthy hair is not only a pleasure for others to see; it's a pleasure to have—even show off. Our hair says a lot about who we are and how we're feeling. In fact, when someone makes a drastic change in her hair, we wonder if she is the same person. Maybe that's why it was so disturbing when Britney Spears shaved her head. Or when Faith Hill chopped off her long blonde curls and got a trendy, razor-cut, bottle blonde style. In fact, when actress Keri Russell cut her long ringlets in favor of a short crop, viewers stopped watching her top-rated show, "Felicity"!

We all want thick, healthy hair that looks shiny and fresh. The best way to get great hair is to grow it. While this chapter does include information about taking care of the hair you have, the real story is the hair you are *going* to have in about six months. Starting today, you are going to grow your own lovely, lustrous locks—then treat them gently so your hair stays full and fabulous.

How Healthy, Luxuriant Hair Grows

Just like your skin, your hair reflects your nutritional status. Behind great hair is great nutrition. There are no hair products that can be applied on the outside that will make up for poor nutrition, and there's a limit to how much conditioners can help damaged hair. Unlike your skin, hair can't repair itself, so if your hair has become thin or brittle, it's time to switch your focus from buying expensive hair products to growing a new head of healthier hair from the inside out.

After you start my Beauty Diet, it usually takes two to three months to start seeing results in the condition of your hair. Scalp hair generally grows at a rate of about half an inch per month, or six inches a year, but this growth rate is very individual—yours could be slower or faster. Also, as people age, their rate of hair growth slows. This means patience and consistency are very important as you await your new halo of fresh hair.

Nourish Your Follicles

Hair follicles can be found all over the body, but the highest density of follicles is on the head, which is also where the longest hairs grow. No new follicles are formed after birth. This means you'll want to take care of the follicles you've got. It also means no product can give you more hair than you already have.

The average person has around 120,000 hairs on his or her head. Blondes tend to have more than the average, brunettes are about average, while redheads tend to have a little less than average.

The hair follicles in your scalp are like little pockets. Each hair grows from rapidly dividing cells in a bulb at the base of the follicle. The root of each hair is nourished by the connective tissue around it. Each follicle needs a constant supply of oxygen, nutrients, and moisture to grow hair properly, which is why good circulation in the scalp is important to gorgeous hair.

Each follicle is associated with one or several tiny sebaceous glands that produce sebum. This natural oil softens and protects both the hair and the scalp. It's easier for sebum to travel down long, straight hair, which explains why curly hair tends to be drier. It's important to make sure sebum does not accumulate and clog the follicles, which can cause loss of hair.

Building a Gorgeous Head of Hair, One Strand at a Time

The part of a strand of hair that is visible above the surface of the scalp is called the *shaft*. Each shaft consists of three concentric layers: the cuticle, the cortex, and the medulla.

- The **cuticle** is the tough outside layer that protects the inner sections of the hair. The cuticle is thin and colorless. Damage to the cuticle can make your hair look dull. It also makes the hair more porous, which means it will absorb more humidity.

- The **cortex** is the middle layer of hair. The proteins twisted together inside the cortex give hair its elasticity. The cortex contains the melanin that gives your hair its color. Eumelanin creates brown or black hair, while pheomelanin makes hair appear red. Blonde hair is a result of very low amounts of melanin; the shade of blonde depends on which type of melanin is present. When melanin is no longer produced in the hair root, the hair grows in without pigment and appears gray.
- The **medulla** is the innermost layer of hair. This part of the shaft reflects light, which is why hair looks so different in sunlight.

Feed Your Head

Healthy hair depends on two things:

1. Having a healthy scalp with healthy follicles
2. Giving your body the building blocks it needs to construct strong, lustrous hair shafts

Stunning hair and a healthy scalp require quality protein, healthy fats, clean water, vital vitamins, and mighty minerals—in the correct amounts. If you consume too much of any one thing, you may end up causing more problems than you correct. For example, an excess of some micronutrients can cause you to lose hair. As long as you follow my Beauty Diet, you'll have all the beneficial components you need with no risks and no harmful side effects.

For a Marvelous Mane, Eat Plenty of Protein

Many people assume that good hair care starts with shampoo. In fact, beautiful hair starts with what you eat. Hair is about 97 percent protein, so protein is a good place to begin this discussion.

Your protein intake can have a dramatic effect on the texture of your hair. Without enough protein, your body cannot make new, beautiful hair to replace the hair that has shed. Too little protein can change the texture of your hair. It can result in hair that is dull, dry, thin, brittle, and weak. Not getting enough protein can affect hair color, too. According to Dr. Martha H. Stipanuk, a Cornell University professor who studies the effects of protein malnutrition, if you're consuming less than 7 percent of calories from protein (or less than 26 grams on a 1,500-calorie diet), you can undergo changes in hair pigmentation. You may start to see pale hair or have a band of hair that is a different color.

A main component of hair is keratin, which gives hair its strength and elasticity. Keratin is made up of amino acids, particularly cysteine. It is not necessary to find dietary sources of cysteine, specifically, because it can be synthesized by your body—provided you consume an adequate amount of protein daily.

Eating food from a variety of different protein sources will help ensure you take in adequate amounts of hair-protective amino acids. Among my Top 10 Beauty Foods, the highest amount of protein is found in salmon, yogurt, walnuts, and oysters. Other good sources of protein include fish, shellfish, turkey, chicken, beef, lamb, soybeans, eggs, nuts, and dairy products. (For more information about protein sources, see Chapter 1.)

Obtain Your Omega-3s

Your body needs quality fats to grow hair, since about 3 percent of the shaft is made up of lipids. In addition, fats are needed to build the cell membranes in the skin of your scalp and for the natural oil that keeps your scalp and hair from drying out.

As you saw in the last chapter, a deficiency of essential fatty acids can cause problems like eczema and dermatitis.

BEAUTY MYTH

Mayonnaise Makes Hair Sleek and Glossy

You would think the ingredients in mayonnaise—including eggs, lemon juice, and oil—would help condition hair. However, applying mayonnaise directly to your hair is just a messy, smelly process that is not worth the unconfirmed benefits. No scientific evidence exists to justify using this sandwich staple for sleek hair; it just leaves your hair feeling heavy and is difficult to rinse out. Treating your hair with mayonnaise is effective only if you have head lice, since mayonnaise suffocates them. For healthy, shiny hair, consume a well-balanced diet that is high in omega-3 fatty acids and monounsaturated fats, found in nuts, avocados, and olive oil. Quality fats will help you maintain healthy, glowing skin and shiny, soft hair from the inside out—with no smelly, sticky residue!

These conditions can affect your scalp and give you dandruff. A lack of essential fatty acids can also make your hair dry, brittle, and slow growing.

You are probably getting enough omega-6 fatty acids in your diet already, but you may have what's called a *subclinical deficiency* of omega-3 fatty acids. Among my Top 10 Beauty Foods, salmon, walnuts, and spinach contain omega-3 fatty acids. Other sources include mackerel, herring, sardines, trout, flax, hemp seeds, walnuts, pumpkin seeds, soybeans, and whole grain products.

Water Is Wondrous for Hair

About 12 to 15 percent of hair is water. As you already know from Chapter 2, it's important to drink plenty of clean water for its beauty benefits and for the proper functioning of every system in the body. Every cell, and every hair follicle, needs water. Water is also needed to transport amino acids, vitamins, minerals, and other nutrients to your scalp, keeping the surface of the skin healthy.

Fiber for Toxin-Free Tresses

As you read in Chapter 1, dietary fiber helps make sure food moves through the intestinal tract in a timely manner. This prevents undigested food from hanging around in the intestines for too long, a problem that can prevent nutrients from being absorbed, leading to dull, dry hair.

Dietary fiber also plays a role in eliminating toxins from the body. When food does not exit the body quickly, toxins can build up in the gut. Some skin-care experts believe toxins contribute to scalp and hair problems. Toxins like heavy metals are absorbed into the hair and excreted, which is why hair analysis is used to look for mercury, aluminum, iron, copper, cadmium, lead, arsenic, and nickel.

To be on the safe side, aim for at least 20 to 25 grams of fiber each day. An added bonus is that fiber takes the edge off appetite, which helps you stay slim.

Valuable Vitamins for Strong, Shiny Strands

Many commercial vitamin and mineral preparations claim they will accelerate hair growth, make hair stronger and longer, help prevent hair loss, and so on. If you are eating a balanced diet, these products should not be necessary. In some cases they might even throw off the natural balance among the nutrients found in the food you eat. Following are some vitamins considered important to a healthy scalp and rich, luxuriant locks.

BETA-CAROTENE/VITAMIN A. Vitamin A plays a vital role in the growth and health of cells and tissues throughout the body, including the cells of the scalp and hair. A fat-soluble antioxidant, vitamin A also helps produce and protect the sebum (oil) in the scalp, and a deficiency can cause dandruff. Ironically, an excess of vitamin A (due to supplements) causes hair loss. My favorite way to get enough vitamin A is to consume plenty of beta-carotene, since the body can then synthesize all the vitamin A it needs. Among my Top 10 Beauty Foods, you'll find significant amounts of beta-carotene in sweet potatoes, spinach, kiwi, and tomatoes. You can also add beta-carotene to your diet with foods like pumpkin, carrots, chilies, mangoes, cantaloupe, and apricots. Among my Top 10 Beauty Foods, preformed vitamin A can be found in oysters, yogurt, and salmon. (For more information on vitamin A, see Chapter 7.)

VITAMIN B COMPLEX. Without vitamin B, hair growth slows and the hair shafts produced are weak and brittle. Some B vitamins are believed to help prevent hair loss, some are thought to assist with the production of keratin, and others are said to boost circulation to the scalp. Vitamin B_6 helps create melanin, which gives hair its color. A major player in commercial hair products is biotin (B_7), perhaps because a bona fide deficiency of this vitamin causes hair loss. On the other hand, studies have not demonstrated that people who already have adequate levels of biotin will benefit from ingesting even more. Some shampoos now contain biotin, but it is not certain this ingredient has any useful effect. Vitamins B_6, B_{12}, and folate (B_9) all help to form red blood cells, which bring oxygen to the hair and allow it to grow at a healthy rate. As you have learned already, the B vitamins work together, so a deficiency of any one of them can affect the proper functioning of the whole group. Different foods have different amounts of each B vitamin, so eat a varied diet to obtain all of them. Among my Top 10 Beauty Foods, the best source of thiamine (B_1) and biotin (B_7) is walnuts, the best source of riboflavin (B_2) and pantothenic acid (B_5) is yogurt, the best source of niacin (B_3) is wild salmon, the best source of folate (B_9) is spinach, and the best source of cobalamin (B_{12})—which is available only from animal sources—is oysters. Spinach, walnuts, and salmon are all good sources of pyridoxine (B_6).

BEAUTY MYTH

Lemon Juice Will Lighten Your Hair

True or false? This beauty myth is actually partly true. If you put lemon juice in your hair and stay inside, nothing will happen, even if you use a hair dryer. To get the lightening effect of lemons, work a generous amount of lemon juice into your hair, then go outside in the sun. The UV light will lighten your hair. When lemon juice is applied to your hair, the citric acid in the lemon juice opens up the cuticle. Once the cuticle is open, the hair becomes more sensitive to changes such as sunlight. The combination of the acid in the lemon juice, the oxygen in the air, and the UV rays from the sun results in a bleaching process. The lemon juice acts as a catalyst, so you will see your hair lighten faster. This reaction is called *acid-catalyzed oxidation.*

VITAMIN C. A nutrient superhero, vitamin C is essential to fabulous hair and a healthy scalp. It aids circulation to the skin and maintains the capillaries that support the hair follicles. If you are not eating abundant amounts of vitamin C–rich foods every day, you may not have enough to take care of your lovely locks. In fact, a deficiency of vitamin C can cause hair breakage. Among my Top 10 Beauty Foods, significant amounts of vitamin C are found in blueberries, kiwi, sweet potatoes, spinach, and tomatoes. Vitamin C is also found in foods like peppers, oranges, strawberries, lemons, and broccoli. (For more information on vitamin C, see Chapter 1.)

VITAMIN E. Because it is a fat-soluble antioxidant, vitamin E protects the scalp's natural oils. Vitamin E also works well with other antioxidants to protect lipid membranes. This vitamin has also been reported to improve scalp circulation. Among my Top 10 Beauty Foods, vitamin E can be found in blueberries, kiwifruit, spinach, tomatoes, and walnuts.

Other good sources of vitamin E include wheat germ, sunflower seeds, safflower and sunflower oils, almonds, peaches, prunes, cabbage, asparagus, and avocados. (For more information on vitamin E, see Chapter 3.)

Must-Have Minerals for Lovely, Lustrous Locks

Good things come in small packages. If you've ever opened a blue gift box from Tiffany and Co., you know that a very big box is great . . . but a small box is better!

For fabulous hair, you need certain minerals in tiny amounts. These trace minerals affect everything from the growth rate of your hair to its color and texture—and the ideal way to obtain them is by eating the variety of whole, natural foods included in my Beauty Diet.

IRON. Iron plays a role in hair health because it helps red blood cells carry oxygen to the hair follicles. While anemia is sometimes an undiagnosed cause of hair loss in women, even if you are not clinically anemic, you can experience hair loss simply from not getting enough iron in your diet. It has been well established that women with alopecia (hair loss and baldness) often have low levels of iron in their blood. For these women, supplementary iron helps hair growth. Iron deficiency can also leave you with lusterless, dry, brittle hair. Among my Top 10 Beauty Foods, the best sources of iron are oysters, spinach, and tomatoes. Other animal sources of iron include clams, lean beef, turkey, duck, lamb, chicken, pork, shrimp, and eggs. Good plant sources of iron include soybeans, lentils, beans, and bran. (For more information on iron, see the end of this chapter.) Plant foods contain nonheme iron, which is not as well absorbed as the heme iron in chicken, fish, and lean beef; however, you can enhance your body's ability to absorb nonheme iron by consuming vitamin C in the same meal.

BEYOND THE BEAUTY DIET

The Lifestyle for Lovely, Luxuriant Locks

Follow these guidelines for thick, gorgeous, captivating hair:

- **Get some exercise.** Take some time to exercise daily, if only for a few minutes. Exercise improves the blood flow to your scalp, which hastens the delivery of oxygen and nutrients to hair follicles, which leads to healthier hair.

- **Avoid rapid weight loss.** A harsh truth is that dieting can make your hair fall out! Crash diets often lack proper nutrition, and rapid weight loss in itself is a stress on the body and can also trigger metabolism changes that affect hair growth. If you lose more than 10 percent of your body weight over a couple of months (e.g., more than 15 pounds if you weighed 150), you can lose hair. Additionally, nutritional deficiencies can contribute to increased hair shedding by weakening hair shafts that cause breakage to the hair and slow regrowth.

- **Avoid low-protein diets.** Hair is 97 percent protein. If you are vegan, make sure you are getting enough protein. Diets that are based on eating mostly rice or mostly fruits do not provide enough protein for beautiful hair.

- **If you smoke, quit now.** Smoking creates free radicals, fills your blood with toxins, and interferes with your body's ability to deliver fresh nutrients to your scalp and hair follicles.

- **Don't stress!** Stress is closely linked to hair loss. Chronic stress interferes with abundant blood circulation in the scalp, which restricts the amount of oxygen and nutrients that reaches your hair follicles. Severe stress—either physical or emotional—causes large numbers of hairs to stop growing and to shift into a resting phase. Two to three months later, all the resting hairs begin falling out. The good news is that eventually this hair grows back.

COPPER. In addition to playing a role in the structure of hair shafts, copper is important to the color of your hair. Because copper is essential to the formation of hemoglobin, it also is involved in bringing oxygen to your hair follicles. If you follow my Beauty Diet, you will not need to worry about your copper intake. A deficiency usually comes either from genetic problems or from taking zinc supplements, which can inhibit the absorption of copper in the body.

SELENIUM. Any discussion of healthy hair has to include selenium, because this trace mineral is important to the scalp. Selenium helps keep skin supple and elastic by preventing cellular damage from free radicals. Ironically, too much selenium (selenosis) can cause hair loss. Among my Top 10 Beauty Foods, you'll find significant amounts of selenium in salmon and oysters. Brazil nuts are an extraordinarily good source of selenium. Other selenium-rich foods include tuna, crab, whole wheat bread, wheat germ, garlic, eggs, and brown rice. (For more information on selenium, see Chapter 2.)

SILICON. This element is found in abundance in our environment, although as we continue to deplete minerals from the soil, our consumption of silicon has declined. In the human body, silicon is found in high concentrations in skin and hair. It is important to the health of your scalp, plus it helps strengthen your hair. High-fiber diets contain lots of silicon, which is widely distributed in whole grains. Silicon is also found in bananas, root vegetables, rice, soybeans, and many other foods.

SULFUR. This trace mineral matters because it is present in cysteine, an amino acid that is crucial to hair growth. This means sulfur helps your body create longer, stronger hair. Sulfur is readily available in a wide variety foods, including eggs, meat, fish, dairy products, onions, and garlic.

ZINC. We know zinc is important to terrific tresses and a healthy scalp because low levels of zinc can cause hair loss and even a loss of eyelashes. A zinc deficiency can also cause the scalp to become dry and flaky. As an antioxidant, zinc helps guard against free-radical damage to your scalp (and elsewhere). Many people are deficient in zinc, but taking zinc supplements can throw off your body's natural balance between zinc and copper. Among my Top 10 Beauty Foods, oysters are an extraordinarily good source of zinc, and yogurt is also helpful. Other foods that contain zinc include seafood, beef, lamb, eggs, whole grains, and nuts. (For more information on zinc, see Chapter 3.)

Nutritional Strategies for Taming Dull, Dry, Brittle, Frizzy Hair

If you have healthy, straight, shining hair like Demi Moore or Heidi Klum, congratulations—you're the exception, not the rule! Most women have to use various tips and tricks to persuade their hair to behave.

Unhealthy hair is dull and dry, with breakage and split ends. Hair that lacks moisture is lightweight, which makes it unmanageable and flyaway. Short, broken strands escape any attempt to control them. If your hair is curly as well as frizzy, you could have a cloud of fuzzy hair instead of gleaming strands. If you suffer from dry, frizzy hair, be sure to check out my Beauty Diet Rx for nutritional solutions to bad hair days.

Gray Hair: Love It or Leave It?

When my friend Rachel discovered her first gray hair, she shrieked—then immediately got her tweezers and plucked

THE BEAUTY DIET RX

For Dry, Brittle Hair

If you are eating an adequate diet, you are probably getting a sufficient amount of protein, plus enough of the trace minerals like copper, sulfur, selenium, and silicon. In addition to following the lifestyle for lovely locks and the maintenance tips for healthy hair discussed in this chapter, you'll want to do the following:

- Get plenty of iron for building strong hair shafts.
- Drink lots of water to help keep your hair hydrated from the inside out.
- Consume more omega-3 fatty acids. Your scalp needs quality fats to produce the sebum that keeps your hair under control.
- Include beta-carotene-rich foods in your diet. From beta-carotene, your body can synthesize vitamin A to keep your scalp healthy.
- Consume plenty of B vitamins, which help keep hair from becoming weak and brittle. They all work together, so eat many different foods to make sure you get enough of each.
- Consume lots of vitamin C–rich foods.
- Focus on foods rich in zinc to keep your scalp healthy and to help hair growth.
- Include vitamin E–rich foods in your diet to protect the lipids in your scalp from free-radical damage.

it out. This approach is working for the time being, but the time will come when Rachel—and the rest of us!—will have to decide whether or not to go gray. She may choose to embrace her gray hair as a sign of her wisdom and experience, or she may say "To heck with that idea!"

The best way to avoid gray hair is to pick parents who have genes for long-lasting hair color. Every person is programmed to develop gray (nonpigmented) hair by a certain age, and no amount of nutritional intervention can change that. However, there are some conditions that can cause hair to turn gray earlier, or more rapidly, than normal. Correcting those processes can help you keep your natural color longer.

THE BEAUTY DIET RX

For Gray Hair

- Correct any underlying health conditions, such as thyroid disorders, that could be making your hair gray. Your hair may grow back in its normal color after you are well.
- Correct any digestive problems you may have, which could be interfering with your ability to absorb nutrients.
- Include an adequate amount of protein in your diet to support the color and texture of your hair.
- Consume an adequate amount of vitamin B_{12} (see Chapter 2).
- If you smoke, stop.
- Relax! Chronic stress will age you, and your hair, prematurely.

When we are young, cells called *melanocytes* produce the pigment that gives our hair its color. Gray hair is caused by a decrease in the functioning of the melanocytes. This is often associated with age but can occur for other reasons. Thyroid disorders may make hair turn gray early, and smoking and stress have been linked to prematurely gray hair.

A link between nutrition and gray hair is vitamin B_{12}. A deficiency of B_{12} can cause gray hair. It's unlikely for most Americans to have a B vitamin deficiency due to a poor diet (though vegans need to supplement their diet with B_{12}), but it can happen if you have problems absorbing nutrients, such as older adults with decreased stomach acid or those with gastrointestinal disorders.

Nutrition to Fight Hair Loss

Today women can be beautiful with or without hair on their heads. When Robin Roberts of the TV show "Good Morning America" lost her hair due to chemotherapy, she walked the runway at an Isaac Mizrahi fashion show completely bald— and she looked sensational doing it!

THE BEAUTY DIET RX

To Fight Hair Loss or Thinning Hair

- Follow the nutritional guidelines for growing healthy hair; the lifestyle tips for lovely, luxuriant locks; and the healthy hair maintenance tips in this chapter.
- If your iron status is questionable, load up on iron-rich foods (see the sidebar on iron at the end of this chapter). Also consider cooking in iron pots.
- Make sure you are getting an adequate amount of protein and zinc in your diet each day. .
- Take a multivitamin to ensure adequate intake of vitamins and minerals, however, be careful with supplements. Occasionally hair loss is caused by oversupplementing with individual vitamins or minerals.
- Avoid losing a lot of weight suddenly.
- Drink my beauty beverage, green tea. Some studies have shown that green tea may influence the serum levels of certain hormones that are linked to at least one form of hair loss, androgenic alopecia, which is common in women and men.

Hair loss ranges from extensive and permanent (going bald) to mild and temporary (hair thinning). Genes have a great deal to do with hair loss, as do hormonal shifts. For example, while you are pregnant, the percentage of hair on your head that is in the growing phase goes up dramatically. After childbirth, more follicles than usual enter the hair's resting phase all at once. When hair cycles all at once, it all falls out at the same time. This can be alarming, but it is completely normal. Fortunately you still have the same number of functioning hair follicles, and the hairs rebalance their phases in a few months at most. While your hair is growing in, it will be thinner than usual, but this is temporary. A similar syndrome can occur after you stop taking birth control pills or switch types of birth control pills.

Iron's Role in Beauty

Recommended Dietary Allowance

WOMEN	MEN
18 mg (ages 19 to 50)	8 mg (ages 19 and above)
8 mg (ages 51 and above)	

As you probably know by now, iron is a key beauty nutrient. The mineral plays important roles in the health of your hair and nails. There are two types of dietary iron: *heme* (derived from animal foods) and *nonheme* (derived from plant foods). The heme variety is easier to absorb; your body will take in up to 35 percent of the iron from animal sources. The nonheme variety is more difficult to absorb; your body takes in only 2 to 20 percent of the iron from plant sources. Vitamin C enhances your absorption of nonheme iron, while calcium can decrease it.

Five Good Whole-Food Sources of Heme (Better-Absorbed) Iron

1. Chicken liver, cooked, 3½ oz.	12.8 mg
2. Oysters, 6 cooked	4.5 mg
3. Beef, chuck, lean, braised, 3 oz.	3.2 mg
4. Clams, cooked, ¾ cup	3.0 mg
5. Turkey, light meat, roasted, 3½ oz.	1.6 mg

Five Good Whole-Food Sources of Nonheme (Harder-to-Absorb) Iron

1. Soybeans, boiled, 1 cup	8.8 mg
2. Lentils, boiled, 1 cup	6.6 mg
3. Blackstrap molasses, 1 tablespoon	3.5 mg
4. Spinach, fresh, boiled, drained, ½ cup	3.2 mg
5. Raisins, ½ cup	1.5 mg

In addition to age and hormone shifts, causes of thinning hair include:

- Too much styling, straightening, curling, coloring, or blow-drying. Hair loss due to overly tight hairstyles is called *traction alopecia.*
- Physical damage to the follicles, such as burning or scarring
- Illness (such as anemia or thyroid disease) or infection (including fungal infections)
- Disorders that interfere with the body's ability to digest food and absorb vital nutrients
- Dropping pounds quickly and being undernourished
- Some medications (including chemotherapy)
- An autoimmune reaction called *alopecia areata,* in which the body attacks the hair follicles and hair falls out. Total hair loss is called *alopecia areata totalis,* while the loss of all the hair on the body is called *alopecia universalis.*
- Stress, either physical or emotional

Most causes of hair thinning are temporary, so with proper treatment hair will grow in again. Massaging the scalp can help stimulate blood flow to the scalp and may help hair grow in more rapidly.

Expert Advice: Topical Nutrients for Hair

According to Dr. David Kingsley, author of *The Hair-Loss Cure: A Self-Help Guide,* and a hair and scalp specialist in New York City, certain nutrients can help the cosmetic appearance of your hair when used in a shampoo or conditioner. Some products, however, just add "natural" ingredients that do little, if anything, for your hair except increase the price of the product! Here is a list of some beneficial ingredients, according to Kingsley:

- **Collagen** is used as a conditioning agent.
- **Castor oil** is used as a moisturizer in hair conditioners.
- **Olive oil** has conditioning benefits, particularly for very dry, coarse hair.
- **Plant proteins** (wheat proteins) have conditioning and hair-strengthening benefits.
- **Vitamin B₃** (niacin): when applied topically, niacin-based products, such as nicotinic acid, have been shown to improve hair growth in a small study for women when compared to a control group.
- **Vitamin B₅** (panthenol) helps provide moisture to the hair shaft.
- **Vitamin E** (tocopherol acetate), a natural antioxidant, has UV protection properties.

How to Maintain Healthy Hair That Is Full of Bounce and Shine

Like your skin, your hair is exposed to the elements every day. Following are some simple hair care tips that will keep your locks lovely and luxuriant.

- **Shampoo Your Hair Properly.** Combination shampoo/ conditioners are less effective than separate products. Shampoo with warm water to open the pores in your scalp and rinse with cool water. A cool rinse (with either water or vinegar and water combined) will close down the cuticle and add shine. Keep in mind that excessive shampooing can strip minerals and natural oils from the hair.
- **Use Leave-In Conditioner.** This helps reduce frizz by rehydrating your hair during the day. Some conditioners, such as Kiehl's, contain UV filters to protect hair from sun damage.
- **Don't Twist Your Hair to Wring out the Water.** Towel-dry your hair and resist rubbing it or creating any sort of friction. Use

a hand towel and squeeze your hair dry, working your way up from the ends to the roots.

- **Use the Blow Dryer in Moderation.** Blow-drying more than three times a week will damage hair. Try to avoid very hot blow dryers and avoid very hot settings on heated flat irons and curling irons. Air-dry your hair when possible.

- **Wear Your Hair in a Loose, Easy Style.** Avoid tight braids or heavy ponytails—these can create bald spots or wide part lines on scalp. Every time you pull your hair back into a tight ponytail or bun, the pressure breaks hair shafts all along your hairline. The short remnants of broken hair pop up as frizz.

- **Have Your Hair Trimmed Every Six to Eight Weeks.** It won't make your hair grow faster, but it will stop split ends from splitting up the hair shaft.

- **Use Chemicals on Your Hair in Moderation.** Lightening your hair color may make your hair drier and frizzier. The chemicals used for curling or relaxing hair chemically alter the shafts, and long-term use of these chemicals can do irreversible damage to the hair or cause hair loss. Combining processes—for example, getting your hair colored and relaxed at the same time—means double the stress for your hair. Limit hair treatments as much as possible and avoid mixing chemical processes.

Nutrition for Long, Shapely, Strong Fingernails

5

Beauty, to me, is about being comfortable in your own skin.
That, or a kick-ass red lipstick.
    —*Gwyneth Paltrow*

Your fingernails are an essential detail of your appearance. *Essential detail* sounds like an oxymoron, like *jumbo shrimp*, but when you think about it, success always depends on the details. Details can make the difference between chocolate pudding and *pot de crème au chocolat*. Even if you spend six hours getting dressed, a detail like spinach in your teeth can ruin your appearance.

Beautiful fingernails say good things about you. They show that you pay attention to details, that you care about cleanliness, and that you successfully manage your time so you can spend a few minutes on keeping your hands attractive. At the very least, you'll want healthy, smooth, clean fingernails that indicate you care about your personal grooming. You may want crisp, polished nails that show you are a professional, no-nonsense kind of person. Perhaps you would like long, elegant nails that give you an air of glamour or sophistication.

Your fingernails also speak volumes about your health. In their natural state, the shape, color, and strength of your nails can change due to many different health factors. Most important to this discussion: fingernails are a very good indicator of your nutritional status. Problem nails can be a sign that your body is not getting all the nutrients it needs.

A Beautiful, Natural Nail

When you stop to think about fingernails, they make a lot of sense. They provide a tough covering for our sensitive fingertips and extend the capabilities of our hands like little tools at the ends of our fingers.

The fingernail itself is a hard covering made mostly of keratin, the same protein found in skin and hair. The part you see is called the *nail plate*. The skin underneath the nail is called the *nail bed*. Healthy fingernails are pink because of the circulation in the blood vessels of the nail bed.

The skin at the bottom of each fingernail is called the *cuticle*. The cuticle overlaps the nail plate. Be kind to your cuticles, because underneath them is the fingernail factory called the *matrix*. New cells for your nails are produced in the matrix. As they grow, they push the older cells out toward the ends of your fingers. This process squashes the older cells so they become hard and flat, forming your fingernails. Unlike your hair, which grows in stages, fingernails are constantly growing.

BEAUTY MYTH

Those White Spots on Your Nails Are Due to Calcium Deficiency

White spots on the fingernails (scientific name: *leukonychia*) are extremely common and harmless. Usually they are caused by trauma to the nail—for example, you bumped your finger without noticing. Temporary injury to the cuticle—for example, pushing it back too roughly—also can cause a white area in the nail that becomes apparent as it grows out. Slamming a car door on your fingers, a rough manicure, or excessive nail biting can result in white spots. Since a normal fingernail takes months to grow out, you may not notice the white spots until some months have passed since you unknowingly hurt your nail.

If you have noticeable white spots or bands on all of your digits, it could be a sign of a zinc, protein, or calcium deficiency. Sometimes nails that appear white accompany disease states, such as cirrhosis of the liver. However, white spots are rarely the first signs of such conditions and usually appear once major symptoms have already occurred.

The white half-moon shape at the bottom of each fingernail is called the *lunula*. The skin that surrounds your fingernails on all three sides is called the *nail folds*. Sometimes the nail folds become swollen or irritated.

You can expect your nails to grow about a tenth of an inch each month. If you're waiting for your nails to grow out, you'll have to be patient. It takes about six months to grow a complete fingernail, but the rate is very individual. Fingernails grow faster when you are young, and they grow more quickly on your dominant hand (if you are right-handed, the fingernails on your right hand grow faster).

The ideal fingernail is strong and resilient—tough but not hard. Natural fingernails should be able to bend instead of break. If you leave the edges alone so they grow out straight, the fingernail will be stronger—plus you'll be less likely to get an ingrown nail.

Growing Your Own: Nourishing Your Nails

Healthy fingernails are pink, firm, and somewhat lustrous. They do not have any strange tint or color. They do not have ridges, pits, white marks, or dark lines. If your fingernails look strange—discolored, clubbed, thick, or with pronounced lines or indentations—this may be a sign of illness. If your fingernails look basically normal but are dry or brittle, this may be a sign that you are not optimally nourished. Your nails may not be getting enough nutrients if you are a super-picky eater, you go on crash diets, or you do not properly digest foods and absorb nutrients.

Recent studies have shown that the health of your nails correlates with the strength of your bones. Women with osteoporosis have less protein in their fingernails. If your diet does not include enough protein and other nutrients to grow strong fingernails, you may have other, less visible problems as well, like weakened bones.

If you already have an excellent diet, adding nutrients will not help your nails. If your diet has room for improvement, now is your chance to reverse any nutritional issues you may have. Although companies market dozens of dietary supplements that are supposed to enhance the growth of your nails, I would much rather have you try my Beauty Diet, which provides you with a wide spectrum of nutrients without any danger of side effects. The Beauty Diet can offer you strong, beautiful, healthy nails in six months—plus, eating well to take care of your nails will help make your whole body strong and gorgeous!

Nail-Boosting Nutrients

Following are the major components of a nail-boosting diet:

WATER. If you have been reading this book from the beginning, you already know that water is a true beauty beverage, as it supports every process and every system in the body. A quick, nonscientific test for dehydration is to press on a fingernail and wait to see how quickly the nail bed returns to pink (from white). If the fingernail doesn't return to its usual pinkish color in less than two seconds, this could be a sign of dehydration. Over the long term, dehydration can make your nails brittle. Make sure you drink enough water to keep all of your cells plump and moist.

PROTEIN. A protein deficiency can show up as white bands across all of your nails. Fingernails are composed mostly of protein, so to grow long, strong, attractive nails you must eat some quality protein every day. As you read in the last chapter, keratin—the main component of hair and fingernails—is made of amino acids, particularly cysteine. However, this does not mean you need supplemental cysteine. Eating a variety of different protein sources will help ensure you take in adequate amounts of amino acids for growing fabulous fingernails. Among my Top 10 Beauty Foods, the highest amount of protein is found in salmon, yogurt, walnuts, and oysters. Other good sources of protein include fish, shellfish, turkey, chicken, beef, lamb, soybeans, eggs, nuts, and dairy products. (For more information about protein sources, see Chapter 1.)

VITAMIN B COMPLEX. The B vitamins include thiamine (B_1), riboflavin (B_2), niacin (B_3), pantothenic acid (B_5), pyridoxine (B_6), biotin (B_7), folic acid/folate (B_9), and cobalamin (B_{12}). While rare, deficiency of vitamin B_{12} can cause hyperpigmentation of the nail plate. The B vitamins work together in the body and are vital to many different processes, including good circulation and cell growth. There are studies indicating that supplemental biotin can strengthen nails, but the articles do not clarify whether the participants started out with an underlying deficiency of biotin. It makes sense that giving biotin to people who are deficient would help their fingernails. If you already consume plenty of B vitamins—

which are readily available in many foods—you probably don't need extra biotin. Among my Top 10 Beauty Foods, the best source of thiamine (B_1) and biotin (B_7) is walnuts, the best source of riboflavin (B_2) and pantothenic acid (B_5) is yogurt, the best source of niacin (B_3) is wild salmon, the best source of folate (B_9) is spinach, and the best source of cobalamin (B_{12})—which is available only from animal sources—is oysters. Spinach, walnuts, and salmon are all good sources of pyridoxine (B_6).

CALCIUM. Nails contain calcium, albeit at a much lower concentration than our bones do. Most Americans, particularly women, do not get enough calcium. While there is no scientific evidence that calcium intake significantly alters nail quality, individuals taking calcium supplements sometimes comment that their nails are less brittle or smoother, or that they grow faster, according to an article published in the *New England Journal of Medicine*. Among my Top 10 Beauty Foods, the best sources of calcium are yogurt, sweet potatoes, and spinach. Good sources of absorbable calcium include milk products, most types of tofu, some dark green leafy vegetables, turnip greens, and canned fish such as salmon and sardines that include bones. (For more information, see Chapter 6.)

IRON. If you are not getting enough iron, your fingernails will show it. Iron-deficiency anemia—which is not uncommon in women—makes nails brittle. If this could be your problem, eat more iron-containing foods. Among my Top 10 Beauty Foods, the best sources of iron are oysters, spinach, and tomatoes. Other animal sources of iron include clams, lean beef, turkey, duck, lamb, chicken, pork, shrimp, and eggs. Good plant sources of iron include soybeans, lentils, beans, and bran. (For more information, see Chapter 4.) You can enhance your body's ability to absorb nonheme iron by consuming vitamin C in the same meal.

THE BEAUTY DIET RX

For Fabulous Fingernails

- Drink plenty of water to hydrate your fingernails from the inside out.
- Consume quality protein every day.
- Make sure you are consuming an adequate amount of B vitamins.
- Consume at least three servings of calcium-rich foods daily.
- Eat lots of foods that contain iron and zinc.
- Avoid crash diets and don't make your diet too restrictive!

ZINC. This essential mineral is found in almost every cell and plays many roles in the body. A deficiency of zinc can cause changes in nails, including white spots or lines, to appear across all of your fingernails at the same time. When I was researching this chapter, I was pleased to come across an online testimonial from someone who said she finally got rid of the white spots in her nails by eating oysters—one of my Top 10 Beauty Foods and a fantastic source of zinc! Yogurt is another of my Top 10 Beauty Foods that contains zinc. Other zinc-rich foods include seafood, beef, lamb, eggs, whole grains, and nuts. (For more information, see Chapter 3.)

Practical Tips to Protect Your Tips

Nail care can be as simple and affordable—or as complex and expensive—as you want it to be. When it comes to keeping your nails in chic shape, a few good habits go a long way.

DO

1. Use moisturizer! Every time you immerse your hands in water, your nails swell. As they dry, they shrink again. This repeated swelling and contracting stresses your nails and can make them brittle and fragile. Whenever your hands get

wet, lightly dry them off and apply moisturizer while they are still a bit damp. The lubricant will seal in the moisture and prevent the cuticles from drying out. Also, apply moisturizer regularly throughout the day. Unpolished nails are permeable, so smooth the lotion all over your hands. Massage the moisturizer into each cuticle to bring circulation to the nail matrix. For a deep treatment, slather your hands liberally with a lotion or oil of your choice before you go to bed, then put on a pair of cotton gloves and leave them on while you sleep.

2. Trim nails after you bathe, while they are soft. Dry nails are more likely to crack when cut.

3. Keep unpolished nails short. They will be less apt to break.

4. Wear rubber gloves when you're gardening, doing the dishes, using cleansers, and so on. To give your nails extra protection, stuff a cotton ball into the fingertip of each glove.

5. Wear mittens (or gloves) outside when it's cold.

6. Deal with nail damage right away. If the edge of a nail gets chipped, file it off before it has a chance to create a bigger problem. Carry an emery board with you, and smooth the rough spot at the first sign of trouble. Always file in the same direction.

DON'T

1. Soak your hands in water if you have a choice.

2. Sabotage your nails by biting them, pulling at the cuticles, or peeling off the polish.

3. Let your hands come in contact with harsh chemicals. Household cleaning products, detergents, and even nail polish removers can weaken and dry out nails.

4. Cut your cuticles. According to nail expert Paul Kechijian, M.D., cuticles are meant to attach tightly to the nail for a waterproof seal. If you break the seal, you lose protection and may get an infection. Don't push your cuticles all the way back!

5. Let your cuticles get so dry that they crack. That's an opportunity for infection to develop.

BEYOND THE BEAUTY DIET

Plain or Polished?

If you truly want to grow out your own long, strong nails, you might consider letting them go *au naturel*. Nail hardeners can "bulletproof" the plates of your nails by reinforcing them with a stiff outer layer, but they can't actually fortify your fingernails. No coating product can penetrate inside the nail to strengthen it. If you have brittle or weak nails that you want to improve, a nail hardener that contains formaldehyde or toluene could end up drying out your nails even more, which is the last thing you need. The real solution for strong, healthy nails comes from the inside, with a little external assistance in the form of cuticle cream or moisturizer. Don't put polish on your nails if you want to be able to moisturize them from the outside. Also, don't polish your nails if it is important for you to avoid toxic chemicals (for example, you are pregnant).

If you choose to polish your nails, do not use nail polish remover more than once a week, because it is drying. If your nail polish chips before then, just do a touch-up instead of using polish remover and starting over. Use an acetone-free nail polish remover, which may be less drying to your nails.

6. Use your nails to open packages, open tabs on soda cans, scratch at stubborn spots, and so on.

Expert Advice: Artificial Nails

Nail expert Paul Kechijian, M.D., is a dermatologist in Great Neck, New York. He was formerly associate clinical professor of dermatology at New York University Medical Center. Following are his thoughts on artificial nails.

Many people wear artificial nails without any problems. Sometimes, however, the glue can cause a facial rash or contact dermatitis of the nail. Usually this doesn't injure the nail bed, but rarely, if it's a bad reaction, nails can be lost permanently. One problem with artificial nails is that you have to soak them in acetone to loosen the glue and get them off. The acetone will dry out the cuticles and the nail, which can make nails more brittle. Also, as the false nail is pulled off, tiny pieces of the nail may go with it. Over several months, you are tearing the surface of the nail and making it more brittle. If you want acrylic fingernails, pick a reputable salon and make sure the salon uses the correct adhesive.

Common Nail Problems

Have you ever met a "parts model"? When you see an ad in a magazine with a pair of hands holding a jar of cuticle cream—those hands are hers. When you see an ad on television with a pair of hands caressing a man's shaved cheek—those are also hers. If you do meet one, you might notice that she is wearing elbow-length gloves year-round as part of her beauty regimen.

I don't recommend wearing elbow-length gloves, but I should point out that most nail problems are caused by trauma (for example, shutting your hand in a cabinet door) or exposure to water and chemicals. If your fingernails look pink and healthy but are brittle or chipped, you probably are being too hard on your hands.

If your diet is good, but your nails are discolored or look strange, they may be trying to tell you something about your health. No one would base a diagnosis strictly on the appearance of your fingernails, but viewed in the context of other signs and symptoms, they can add information that helps complete the diagnostic puzzle. Remember to mention your fingernails when you visit the doctor, as their color, shape, texture, and markings may all give clues to underlying illness.

BEAUTY MYTH

Eating Gelatin Strengthens Nails

Gelatin is a good source of protein, and protein is the main component of nails. So it may make sense to eat more gelatin products for healthier nails. However, no evidence proves that consuming gelatin can help your nails grow. Amino acids are the building blocks of protein, and they are used by all parts of the body. Your body has no way of knowing that you are hoping something you eat—for example, gelatin—will be used exclusively for your fingernails. Unless you are deficient in protein, which is uncommon in the United States, consuming extra protein supplements or applying protein-based products on your nails won't help your nails become stronger. To have healthy, strong nails, follow my Beauty Diet, which includes adequate protein and other nutrients—and wear gloves when necessary!

Nutrition for a Gleaming, White, Healthy Smile

6

I've never seen a smiling face that was not beautiful.
—*Anonymous*

Nothing is more attractive than a healthy smile. Do you remember the television show "The Swan"? The series would start with a group of women who were at a point in their lives when they could really use a makeover. Every aspect of their appearance was improved, and the contestants were not allowed to see themselves in a mirror until the dramatic unveiling of their new look. Ultimately the woman who experienced the biggest transformation from ugly duckling was voted "the swan."

The "Swan" contestants underwent procedures from head to toe, including expensive hair treatments, nose jobs, and breast implants, not to mention new clothes and makeup. But what often made the biggest difference of all was the cosmetic dental work they received. Many got flawless white veneers for their teeth, giving them sensational celebrity smiles.

The great thing about a fabulous smile is that it always looks terrific. If you pushed Julia Roberts into a swimming pool, her hair would go flat, her makeup would run, and her clothes would get soggy, but she would still be camera-ready with her million-dollar smile. When you have a healthy grin, it's with you from the moment you wake up in the morning until your last good-night kiss.

At a cost upward of a thousand dollars per tooth, most of us can't afford perfect veneers, but there is a great deal we can do to take care of the teeth nature gave us. In addition to proper oral care, it comes down to the choices we make about the food we put in our mouths.

Tooth Anatomy: Speak Like a Dentist

The visible part of each tooth is called the *crown*. The crown is covered with enamel, which is translucent and white. Even though enamel is the hardest substance in the body, it can be eaten away by decay. The stronger your enamel is, the more resistant it is.

The root of the tooth is below the gum line. It makes up about two-thirds of the tooth and holds the tooth in place because it is embedded in bone. Roots are covered with cementum, which helps attach teeth to the alveolar bone (jawbone). Between the cementum and the bony socket of the jawbone there is a cushioning layer called the *periodontal ligament*.

Under the enamel and cementum of each tooth is the dentin, which is yellow, porous, and harder than bone. Sometimes the color of the dentin shows through the enamel, making teeth look yellow.

At the center of the tooth is the pulp, which contains blood vessels and nerves. The pulp nourishes the dentin and is essential to the health of the tooth.

The gums, or gingiva, are the soft tissue around the base of the teeth. The tooth and gums meet at the gum line. Sometimes debris builds up along the gum line, which causes problems.

Saliva is crucial to healthy teeth. Saliva maintains the correct pH level in the mouth, and it contains trace minerals to help maintain the enamel of your teeth.

Watch Your Mouth: How Common Problems Develop

Beauty and health are always closely related, but when it comes to an attractive smile, they are inseparable. Ugly teeth are an immediate turnoff, which is why we associate them with pirates and witches.

The two essential components of a beautiful smile are strong teeth and healthy gums. You're in luck, because my Beauty Diet can help you preserve both. I need to take just a minute to explain how problems develop so you'll see why making changes in your diet can give you a shining smile.

Tooth Troubles You Don't Want

Every day a sticky film of bacteria called *plaque* forms on your teeth. The bacteria in plaque thrive on sugar and starches from the food you eat and produce acids that over time can destroy the enamel of your teeth, creating holes that are called *cavities* or *caries*.

Each time you eat food that contains sugars or starches, your teeth are attacked by decay-causing acids for 20 minutes or longer. Anything that keeps the environment of the mouth acidic—for example, eating acidic foods frequently or exposing your teeth to stomach acid from acid reflux problems, vomiting, or bulimia—can contribute to dental erosion.

We've all heard that sugar is bad for teeth, and some of us may even have had our Halloween candy hidden away by our parents, who wanted to keep our smiles bright. Although candy is harmful to teeth, snacks like potato chips and cookies are even worse. Simple sugars are relatively easy to wash away, but food particles from starches tend to get lodged in between our teeth, providing a carbohydrate feast for plaque.

Brushing and flossing are essential because they remove the film of plaque around and in between your teeth. If plaque is allowed to remain on your teeth for too long, it mineralizes and turns into a hard accumulation called *tartar*. You can't brush away tartar; it can be removed only by your dentist or hygienist.

Gum Disease: Not a Fun Disease

Plaque that has built up along the gum line also can irritate your gums, leading to gingivitis, which is characterized by puffy, red, bleeding gums. At this stage the inflammation is mild, and the supporting structures that hold your teeth in place have not been affected—yet.

If gingivitis is not treated, plaque can move below the gum line and spread to the roots of the teeth. Now the problem is called *periodontitis*. Plaque begins to damage the fibers and bone that keep your teeth in position. It also can force your teeth to separate from your gums, creating pockets where bacteria can hide. Sometimes your teeth will look healthy even though gum disease is developing where you can't see it. Bad breath for no obvious reason can be a sign of periodontitis. Treating periodontitis can be an unpleasant process, but it prevents further damage to your teeth.

The final stage of gum disease, *advanced periodontitis*, is not pretty. By this time the fibers and bone supporting your teeth have been destroyed. The teeth start to shift and loosen and may need to be pulled. In fact, periodontal disease is the leading cause of tooth loss in adults 35 and older.

Women may be more susceptible to periodontitis because of their hormones. Women are more prone to the development of periodontal disease during puberty, at certain points in their monthly menstrual cycle, when they are taking birth control pills, while they are pregnant, and at menopause. In addition to oral contraceptives, certain drugs can make you more vulnerable to gum disease, including some antidepressants and some heart medications, due to dry mouth.

Poor nutrition—the combination of eating foods that harm the teeth, plus not getting enough nutrients—can cause gum disease to progress faster and become more severe. My Beauty Diet will provide all the nutrients you need to protect your health and nourish every part of your natural beauty, including your sexy smile.

Healthy Eating Habits to Protect Your Pearly Whites

There's a difference between "diet" and "nutrition," although for practical purposes you can't separate the two. Your diet is whatever foods you eat. Your nutrition comes from your diet. This chapter is a little different from the others, because when it comes to maintaining the health of your teeth and gums, your food choices have both short-term effects and long-term nutritional consequences.

The foods you eat immediately affect what is going on in your mouth. For example, if you snack on potato chips, the food particles that get stuck in your teeth become food for plaque, and bacteria will start munching on your teeth for the next 20 minutes or so. Your hair and skin won't suffer—

but your teeth might. If you eat potato chips every afternoon and night at the expense of other nutrient-rich foods, your teeth and gums, as well as other aspects of your health, may suffer.

Nutrients That Nourish Your Teeth and Gums

Teeth are built to last. When you were a kid, you probably were taught that brushing, flossing, and visiting the dentist would be enough to keep your teeth and gums healthy. Today health-care professionals know this is no longer enough, because nutrition plays a huge role in maintaining an attractive smile. If you brush and floss regularly, make regular trips to the dentist, *and* get the right nutrients from your diet, you should be able to use your teeth for a hundred years. Following are some of the major nutrients you'll need to keep your teeth and gums healthy and bright.

CALCIUM. Most people realize that children need calcium to build their adult teeth. From there they assume that by the time adult teeth come in they are "finished." The truth is that adult teeth still need calcium and other trace minerals to make them more resistant to decay. We also need calcium to support the health of the alveolar bone. Statistics indicate people with healthy calcium levels have significantly lower rates of periodontal disease, while low calcium intake is associated with higher rates of periodontal disease. All of my Top 10 Beauty Foods contain at least trace amounts of calcium, but the best source is plain low-fat yogurt, with 448 milligrams in a cup (about half your recommended dietary allowance). Other good sources of calcium include dairy products, Chinese cabbage, and sardines.

VITAMIN D. This vitamin is necessary for the absorption of calcium. Vitamin D is not found in very many foods, which is why commercial milk, cereals, and other foods are fortified with it. You can synthesize your own by sunbathing, but

Calcium's Role in Beauty

Recommended Dietary Allowance

WOMEN	MEN
1,000 mg (ages 19 to 50)	1,000 mg (ages 19 to 50)
1,200 mg (ages 51 and above)	1,200 mg (ages 51 and above)

Calcium is the most abundant mineral in the body. More than 99 percent of the body's calcium is in the bones and teeth, where the mineral provides beauty-boosting benefits. The remaining 1 percent is found throughout the body.

Good sources of absorbable calcium include most milk products, most types of tofu, some dark green leafy cabbage family vegetables, turnip greens, and canned fish such as salmon and sardines that include bones. Moderately good calcium sources include ice cream and most green leafy vegetables. Cream cheese and cottage cheese contain calcium, but not nearly as much as other types of cheese.

10 Good Whole-Food Sources of Calcium

1. Yogurt, nonfat, plain, 1 cup	448 mg
2. Ricotta cheese, part-skim, ½ cup	337 mg
3. Sardines, canned in oil, 3 oz.	324 mg
4. Milk, fat-free, 1 cup	316 mg
5. Mozzarella cheese, part-skim, 1.5 oz.	310 mg
6. Swiss cheese, 1 oz.	272 mg
7. Salmon with bones, 3 oz.	205 mg
8. Turnip greens, cooked, 1 cup	200 mg
9. Cheddar cheese, low-fat, 1 oz.	118 mg
10. White beans, ½ cup	96 mg

sun exposure prematurely ages the skin and carries the risk of skin cancer. Among my Top 10 Beauty Foods, vitamin D is found in salmon and oysters. Other good sources include fortified milk, cod liver oil, and sardines (for more information, see Chapter 2).

MAGNESIUM. Magnesium is a major component of teeth and bones. This mineral works together with calcium and plays many other important roles in the body. Spinach, walnuts, and dark chocolate, three of my Top 10 Beauty Foods, all contain magnesium.

VITAMIN C. We know a deficiency of vitamin C (scurvy) loosens teeth and causes bleeding and swelling in the gums. Vitamin C is extremely important to the health of your mouth, not only for its antioxidant properties but also because it helps maintain and repair connective tissue. This multitasking vitamin is essential for the formation of collagen, which helps keep your gums healthy. Without vitamin C, gums and the connective tissues holding teeth begin to erode. In a study involving more than 12,000 U.S. adults conducted at the State University of New York at Buffalo, people who consumed the lowest amounts of vitamin C were at the greatest risk for gum disease. Vitamin C also enhances immune function and promotes healing. Among my Top 10 Beauty Foods, you'll find significant amounts of vitamin C in kiwi, blueberries, sweet potatoes, spinach, and tomatoes. You can also get your daily dose of vitamin C from foods like peppers, oranges, strawberries, lemons, and broccoli (for more information, see Chapter 1).

OMEGA-3 FATTY ACIDS. Omega-3s are helpful to gum health because they help reduce inflammation and support bone health. A study published in *Clinical Nutrition* concluded that alveolar bone destruction in periodontal disease is associated with an imbalance between the omega-6 and omega-3 fatty acids and that it makes sense to treat gum disease by increasing omega-3s in the diet because this will shift the body away from the production of arachidonic acid and inflammation-boosting prostaglandins. Among my Top 10 Beauty Foods, you can obtain omega-3 fatty acids from salmon, spinach, and walnuts. (For more information on essential fatty acids, see Chapter 1.)

Eight Tips for Beautiful Teeth

The following eight eating habits will make sure you never have to hide your winning smile.

1. Condense Your Consumption of Carbs

My brother Jeff, an orthodontist, recently asked me, "Which do you think is more harmful to your teeth: having a piece of chocolate cake at one sitting or sipping a cup of coffee with sugar throughout the day?" Believe it or not, the answer is the coffee, because sipping continuously throughout the day provides a constant opportunity for the sugars to attack your teeth (chances are, we eat a piece of chocolate cake pretty quickly!).

Teeth don't really care about portion control. For them, eating one caramel has basically the same effect as eating 20. However, for your teeth, timing is everything. Eating 20 caramels all at once is better for your teeth than eating one caramel every so often, all day. Sucking on hard candy or nibbling on chips and cookies all day nourishes bacteria and bathes teeth with acids that cause cavities. (For 20 or more minutes, bacteria feed off the carbohydrates, and the acids produced go to work on your teeth until your saliva is able to wash away the food particles and neutralize the acids.) If you snack, eat every three to four hours, not every three to four minutes!

- **Bad for teeth** are lollipops, cough drops, peppermints, and sweet candies that bathe the teeth in sugar. If you tend to eat these sweets in succession, your teeth get a sugar bath all day.
- **Even worse for teeth** are chewy or sticky treats like Starburst candies, Tootsie Rolls, Gummi Bears, caramels, and Skittles. Sticky foods stay on teeth longer, and this increases acid formation.

- **Worst of all for teeth** are soft, sweet, sticky foods like cake, candy, bread, potato chips, crackers, cookies, sugar-coated cereals, cream-filled cookies, and so on. Unlike simple sugars, starchy snacks get stuck in between your teeth and linger in the mouth, continuing to feed the bacteria that cause tooth decay. If you don't brush or floss, food particles may hang around for hours or days.

To discourage tooth decay, condense your consumption of carbs, and avoid sticky, sugary treats!

2. Snack with Care

When you crave a snack, reach for some sugar-free gum with xylitol. It increases the production of saliva, which is your body's natural mechanism for washing away food and neutralizing acid, plus xylitol can temporarily slow the growth of the bacteria that cause tooth decay. If gum won't do the trick, choose among the following smile protectors.

- **Apples.** Personally I love the way a crunchy apple makes my teeth feel. Apples are sweet but not sticky, plus they increase the flow of saliva—your best natural defense against cavities and gum disease.
- **Carrots.** Crunchy vegetables clean and stimulate the gums, helping to scrape away food particles. Foods with fiber have a cleansing effect, and they also stimulate saliva flow, rinsing away bacteria and keeping your mouth hydrated.
- **Cheese.** A small piece of hard cheese is good for your teeth. Cheese has calcium and other trace minerals in it, plus hard cheeses have been shown to generate saliva, which neutralizes the pH level in your mouth. That means your mouth is less acidic and therefore less prone to tooth decay.
- **Cranberries.** Scientists have discovered that cranberries contain a compound that can stop bacteria from clinging to

the teeth, blocking the formation of plaque deposits. However, cranberries are naturally bitter, so foods with cranberries usually have sugar added.

- **Dark chocolate.** This treat offers beauty benefits to our teeth! Researchers have discovered a cocoa extract that is more effective at protecting teeth than fluoride. A substance called *theobromine* helps harden tooth enamel, making teeth less susceptible to decay. Unfortunately, even high-quality dark chocolate is only about 3 percent theobromine, but the substance may soon be appearing in commercial toothpaste.
- **Kiwi.** One of my Top 10 Beauty Foods, kiwi has many beauty benefits and is a good choice for teeth because of its high vitamin C content (see Kiwifruit in Chapter 2).
- **Onions.** Granted, raw onions are not your typical American snack, but they do contain powerful antibacterial compounds that help fight cavities. Adding a few onion slices to your salad or sandwich could hurt your breath but help your teeth.
- **Raisins.** A study at the University of Illinois in Chicago found that raisins contain oleanolic acid, a phytochemical that in lab tests inhibited the growth of the oral bacteria that can lead to poor gum health and cavities. At a concentration of 31 micrograms per milliliter, oleanolic acid prevented *S. mutans* from adhering to tooth surfaces. At 62 micrograms per milliliter, it inhibited the growth of *Porphyromonas gingivalis*, a leading cause of periodontal disease.
- **Sushi with wasabi.** Known as *Japanese horseradish*, wasabi contains isothiocyanates that inhibit the growth of cavity-causing *S. mutans*, according to preliminary research.

3. Avoid Soda—of Any Kind!

In 2003, the average American consumed over 45 gallons of soda per year, according to *General Dentistry* magazine. You might think that lemon-lime sodas are better than colas or that diet soda is better than regular, but the sad truth is that no soda is OK for your teeth.

Most sodas contain huge amounts of glucose, fructose, sucrose, and other simple sugars. As you sip your soda, the bacteria in your mouth dance with joy. The longer you take to finish your drink, the happier they are.

Carbonated soft drinks also contain acids that can harm teeth, such as citric and phosphoric acid. One recent study that rated the effect of 20 different soft drinks on tooth enamel found that diet sodas were less erosive than their sugary cousins, but they were still harmful for teeth. The most erosive sodas in the study were 7Up, Coke, Squirt, Pepsi, and RC Cola. The least harmful were root beer and Diet Coke.

4. Take That Mug off Your Desk

We have a tendency to sip drinks all day. With breakfast, we drink juice. At the office, we may have our own mug by the office coffeepot. On the run, we grab a sports drink. Before a presentation, we drink vitamin water. At a game, we drink soda. At a picnic, we have iced tea. When we start feeling tired, we have a caffeinated drink to stay alert.

All these nonsoda drinks can wreak havoc on your teeth. Sweetened sports drinks, energy drinks, iced teas, and lemonades all feed the bacteria that can cause irreversible damage to your dental enamel. Flavor additives such as malic, tartaric, and other organic acids are aggressive about eroding teeth.

If you must drink something other than water or green tea, use a straw. If you sip acidic drinks through a straw aimed toward the back of your mouth, your teeth are less likely to come into contact with erosive chemicals, which helps preserve the enamel.

5. Watch out for Foods That Stain Your Teeth

The following foods and beverages can stain teeth:

- Coffee
- Tea, iced tea drinks

BEYOND THE BEAUTY DIET

Smoking and Oral Health

There are a thousand reasons to stop smoking, and here is another one: smoking puts you at greater risk of gum disease by interfering with blood flow to the gums. Smoking also is a leading cause of tooth loss, because it disrupts the normal function of gum tissue and the way bone and soft tissue attach to your teeth.

Smoking is associated with brown, stained teeth; bad breath; inflammation of the salivary glands; increased buildup of plaque; increased bone loss from the jaw; delayed healing of oral surgery; and an increased risk of developing cancer.

- Red wine
- Colored juices, such as grape juice and cranberry juice
- Curry
- Cola drinks
- Dark sauces such as soy sauce
- Balsamic vinegar

And, of course, let's not forget the worst culprit of all: smoking, which turns teeth brown.

6. Avoid Dry Mouth

"Dry mouth" sounds a little silly until it happens to you. Considered one of the leading causes of dental disease, dry mouth occurs when you don't have enough saliva to keep your mouth moist, to neutralize acids in your mouth, and to rinse away food particles from between your teeth. Dry mouth is no joke, because it is a leading cause of tooth decay.

Certain medications can cause dry mouth, as can alcohol. Hormonal changes can influence saliva production as well. To keep the inside of your mouth wet, chew sugarless gum and drink more water (as well as green tea—see number 8). A

THE BEAUTY DIET RX

What to Eat (and Drink) for a Sensational Smile

- Keep the inside of your mouth hydrated by drinking water or chewing gum.
- Drink lots of my beauty beverage, green tea.
- Eat plenty of the nutrients you need to nourish your healthy, pink gums and to keep your teeth strong and bright: calcium, vitamin D, magnesium, vitamin C, and omega-3 fatty acids.
- Eat sticky carbohydrates with your main meals, so the particles will get scrubbed off your teeth.
- Choose snacks that wash easily off the teeth.
- Avoid sipping drinks throughout the day. If you must drink something other than water or green tea, use a straw.
- To keep your teeth their whitest, avoid foods that stain.
- Avoid foods that might break your teeth.

glass of water after a meal will help wash away food particles and decay-causing bacteria, but, unlike most beverages, it won't introduce new sugars to your mouth or add calories to your diet. Plus, water can help you feel full and lose weight.

7. Avoid Those Little Bites That Break Teeth

Ice, peanut brittle, and popcorn kernels are all hard on teeth. If your teeth have any weak spots, chomping on something hard could snap off a tooth fragment. Ice and tooth enamel are both crystalline. When you knock two crystals together, the weaker one usually breaks. Sometimes that could be your tooth!

8. Drink More Green Tea

Because green tea is made from unfermented leaves, it contains greater amounts of polyphenols (and less caffeine) than black tea does. Green tea polyphenols prevent plaque from adhering to your teeth and inhibit the growth of the bacteria that can then cause tooth decay. Also, green tea contains natural fluoride, which helps protect tooth enamel from decay.

The Proper Way to Take Care of Your Teeth

Remember, the most important part of good dental hygiene is commitment.

- Brush your teeth twice a day, with fluoride toothpaste. Brush your tongue too.
- There is a proper way to brush teeth. Have your dentist or hygienist show you.
- Use a toothbrush that has soft bristles. Electric toothbrushes can help ensure that you brush for the right amount of time and prevent hard scrubbing, but they aren't necessarily better.
- Replace your brush every three months—and don't share it with anyone! Your toothbrush comes into contact with millions of bacteria in your mouth.
- Floss between your teeth every day. This helps remove plaque and food particles from between the teeth and under the gum line—places where toothbrush bristles can't reach.
- Try brushing and flossing right after dinner while you still have the energy. This also will discourage evening snacking and help you stay slim.
- Use an antimicrobial mouth rinse to inhibit bacterial activity in dental plaque. Some have fluoride, which helps prevent tooth decay.
- Visit your dentist regularly—at a minimum, twice a year. Only your dentist or hygienist can clean the tartar off your teeth and catch little problems before they become big.

BEAUTY MYTH

Brushing with Salt Whitens Teeth

Salt has a coarse texture, which works to thin the outer layer of your teeth, resulting in brighter and whiter teeth. This is not much different from using a scouring pad on your body to soften your skin. Using salt as a treatment for whiter teeth will shift stains, but it comes at a high cost, such as sensitive gums and teeth and the potential for cavities.

Expert Advice: Teeth Whitening

Following is some information on teeth whitening, courtesy of my brother, Dr. Jeff Drayer, a New York–based orthodontist, and the American Dental Association (ADA).

There are many different approaches to whitening teeth, from over-the-counter strips to professional procedures. The difference in the result depends on the levels of active ingredients.

Teeth with a yellowish color tend to whiten well with a bleaching process, whereas teeth that are grayish do not bleach as well. Teeth that are stained due to tetracycline may be very resistant to whitening procedures.

- **Enamel microdermabrasion.** Your dentist can use this procedure to file off localized stains or spots.
- **Whitening mouthwash.** These preparations may contain hydrogen peroxide to bleach your teeth, as well as other ingredients.
- **Whitening toothpaste.** This can make your teeth appear a little lighter by removing stains on the surface of the teeth, but it will not actually bleach your teeth.
- **Over-the-counter tooth-whitening products.** These range from "pens" to whitening strips to trays of gel you put in your mouth. These methods may be helpful for maintenance following a professional procedure.

Magnesium's Role in Beauty

Recommended Dietary Allowance

WOMEN	MEN
310 mg (ages 19 to 30)	400 mg (ages 19 to 30)
320 mg (ages 31 and above)	420 mg (ages 31 and above)

By working together with calcium and vitamin D, magnesium helps to maintain strong, beautiful bones and teeth. Magnesium plays a role in over 300 chemical reactions that occur in the body.

10 Good Whole-Food Sources of Magnesium

1. Spinach, boiled, 1 cup	157 mg
2. Pumpkin seeds, ¼ cup	185 mg
3. Soybeans, cooked, 1 cup	148 mg
4. Salmon, chinook, baked, 4 oz.	138 mg
5. Sunflower seeds, raw, ¼ cup	127 mg
6. Sesame seeds, ¼ cup	126 mg
7. Halibut, baked, 4 oz.	121 mg
8. Black beans, cooked, 1 cup	120 mg
9. Almonds, dry roasted, ¼ cup	99 mg
10. Walnuts, ¼ cup	44 mg

- **Dental trays with gel prescribed by your dentist.** Tooth-whitening kits from the dentist produce faster results because they contain a stronger peroxide bleaching agent than anything you can buy over the counter.
- **One-time in-office treatment.** Your teeth can be whitened by several shades in under an hour, dramatically improving the appearance of your teeth. You may have three applications of whitening gel during one appointment. A special lamp is used to activate the whitening gel and speed up the whitening process. This approach uses a strong whitening agent, so there's more potential for temporary sensitivity.

The ADA advises patients to consult with their dentists to determine the most appropriate treatment to meet their needs.

Nutrition for Clear, Bright, Sparkling Eyes

7

Beauty is how you feel inside, and it reflects in your eyes.
It is not something physical.
—*Sophia Loren*

I f I had to guess, I'd say you probably would be willing to run to the grocery store with your hair quickly pulled back in a ponytail. You most likely would take out the dog wearing your boyfriend's oversized sweatshirt. You might even drop the kids off at school in the morning still wearing your bunny slippers. But leave the house without your eyebrows plucked? Not likely! If you got pinkeye, would you let other people see you without eye makeup—and wearing greasy eye medicine? Only if you could wear dark sunglasses, right? Personally I don't like to do errands without at least some mascara and eyeliner. I never know whom I might see—and who might see me!

You probably spend extra attention on your eyes because they are so expressive. You look into other people's eyes to see if they are telling the truth, to find out what they are feeling, to show them you are fearless, and to let them know you love them. Your eyes not only see the world but also communicate to the world your thoughts, feelings, and intentions.

The way you present your eyes says something too. You may prefer the fresh-faced, minimal-makeup approach, showing that you are a natural beauty. Or you may prefer the ultraglam, richly made-up look, complete with jewel-toned eye shadow and false eyelashes—including, if you're Madonna, $10,000 mink eyelashes with diamonds on them! Part of the beauty of eyes, of course, is that you can have it both ways and simply switch your palette to match your mood.

When you're healthy, your eyes are clear and bright. If you're not feeling well, other people will be able to tell immediately by your eyes. Sometimes the appearance of your eyes gives clues to systemic problems, like liver, thyroid, or kidney disorders. Stunning eyes say so much about you, and they are flattering to your entire look. Following is my best advice for keeping your eyes healthy and bright.

Looking Good and Seeing Well

Our eyes put up with a lot. We expect them to be 100 percent reliable, and we count on them to see accurately under all sorts of conditions, from the deepest night to a day with blazing sun reflecting off white snow. We subject our eyes to all kinds of tasks, from reading the tiny print on medicine bottles and BlackBerrys to scanning the far horizon. As children we read under the covers with flashlights, sat too close to the television, and had flashbulbs go off in our faces so brightly that we saw spots afterward. Now that youth is no longer on our side, it makes sense to give our eyes some extra nutritional support so they will stay clear and captivating.

When we laugh or squint, we get "crow's feet" at the corners of our eyes. Laughing is always beneficial, but squinting . . . not so much. The skin around the eyes is the thinnest on the body, and because it has very few sweat or oil glands, it tends to be dry. With repeated squinting, the wrinkles become more embedded, giving the face more character, but a less youthful appearance. To keep the skin around your eyes flexible and hydrated, use moisturizer and follow my nutritional guidelines for thirsty skin in Chapter 3.

Inside the Eye

The colored part of the eye is the iris—the unique aspect of another person's face that is so memorable. The pupil is the black circle in the middle of the eye that expands in the dark to let in more light and contracts in the sunlight to keep out excessive UV rays.

Behind the iris is the lens. The lens of the eye contains high levels of vitamins C and E, which suggests these are eye-healthy vitamins to include in our diets. The cells of the lens make a special set of proteins called *crystallins* that allow red, blue, green, yellow, and UV wavelengths to pass through the lens and onto the retina. The lens helps to focus light on the retina, which then sends to the brain an image of what we are seeing. The lens of the eye is the only organ that never sheds a cell.

The retina is a light-sensitive membrane that contains millions of light receptor cells. It lines the eye and receives images from the lens. The retina has high concentrations of omega-3 fatty acids; specifically, very high levels of docosahexaenoic acid (DHA) are present in the membranes of photoreceptor cells. The retina also contains zinc, plus high levels of the related carotenoids lutein and zeaxanthin. Lutein, a natural yellow pigment, is highly concentrated in the macula lutea, a yellowish spot close to the center of the retina. Lutein filters out blue light, which is believed to be damaging—hence, lutein has been dubbed *natural sunglasses*. Lutein has antioxidant properties as well. It is not manufactured by the body, so the only way to obtain it is by eating it. Spinach, one of my Top 10 Beauty Foods, is an excellent source of lutein.

Over time, free radicals damage the retina as well as components of the lens, including lipids and proteins. The eyes are protected in part by enzymes that digest damaged proteins. Antioxidants not only help protect the eyes from free-radical damage directly, but also keep the protective enzymes functioning longer.

When damage to the lens accumulates, opaque areas called *cataracts* gradually develop. Different kinds of damage to the retina—for example, problems caused by premature birth, diabetes, or high blood pressure—are grouped under the umbrella term *retinopathy*. When damage to the light-sensitive cells at the back of the retina—more specifically, to the area that produces the sharpest vision, called the *macula*—accumulates over time, the result is called *age-related macular degeneration*, or *AMD*.

Keeping Your Eyes Bright: Nutrition and Age-Related Eye Disorders

Lots of research regarding ophthalmic nutrition has been done, with intriguing results. An early study researched the link between eye health and supplementary vitamin C, vitamin E, beta-carotene, and zinc. This landmark study from the National Eye Institute (part of the National Institutes of Health) was called the Age-Related Eye Disease Study, or AREDS. Participants took high-dose supplements for six years. Scientists concluded the supplements were somewhat protective against macular degeneration, but they did not help restore vision that was already lost.

Some protection against cataracts was apparent in a sub-study of the federally funded Nurses' Health Study called the Nutrition and Vision Project, or NVP. This study showed that women with the highest intakes of vitamin C, vitamin E, riboflavin (vitamin B$_2$), folate (vitamin B$_9$), beta-carotene, lutein, and zeaxanthin had a lower prevalence of opaque areas in the eye. Those who used vitamin C supplements for 10 or more years were 64 percent less likely to have nuclear opacification than those who didn't take vitamin C supplements.

Several studies have examined the link between omega-3 fatty acids and age-related eye problems. A 2007 study from the National Eye Institute concluded that omega-3 fatty acids are protective against retinopathy in mice and suggested that increasing omega-3 fatty acid intake in premature infants may significantly decrease the occurrence of reti-nopathy due to prematurity. Scientists are hoping that, by extension, omega-3 fatty acids will also prove helpful against retinopathy due to diabetes, as well as age-related macular degeneration.

Not everyone agrees that nutritional intervention can help prevent age-related eye disorders. A 2007 article in the *British Medical Journal* reveals that researchers in Australia con-cluded from a meta-analysis of existing studies that the only lifestyle-related risk factor for macular degeneration estab-lished beyond a doubt is smoking. On the flipside, recent research on omega-3 fats is very promising. In June 2008, researchers from Australia concluded that a high dietary intake of omega-3 fatty acids was associated with a 38 percent reduction in the risk of late (advanced) AMD, while eating fish twice a week was associated with a reduced risk of both early and late AMD. The study, published in the *Archives of Ophthalmology*, was a meta-analysis of nine previously published studies, involving a total of 88,974 individuals.

At this point scientists know that oxidative stress damages the tissues of the eye. They have known for a long time that the lens of the eye contains high levels of vitamins C and E, that the retina contains zinc as well as an unusually high concentration of omega-3 fatty acids, and that the yellow color of the macula comes from lutein and zeaxanthin. Common sense suggests that consuming the water-soluble antioxidant vitamin C, the fat-soluble antioxidants vitamin E and beta-carotene, the essential mineral zinc, healthy omega-3 fatty acids, and the related carotenoids lutein and zeaxanthin from my Top 10 Beauty Foods would support eye health.

Nutrition That Keeps Your Eyes Sparkling

You can be an eyesore . . . or you can be eye candy! Clear, vibrant eyes show that you are on top of the world. By following my Beauty Diet, you can protect your beautiful eyes and your precious sight. Here are some specific diet tips to keep your eyes sparkling:

- **Eat plenty of foods rich in fresh vitamin C**, which not only is an eye-protective antioxidant, but also nourishes your natural beauty in countless other ways. Among my Top 10 Beauty Foods, you'll find lots of vitamin C in blueberries, kiwi, sweet potatoes, spinach, and tomatoes. You can increase your daily dose of vitamin C by eating foods like peppers, grapefruit, oranges, strawberries, lemons, and broccoli. (For more information, see Chapter 1.)

- **Eat lots of whole, natural foods that contain the fat-soluble antioxidant vitamin E** to protect the lipids in your lovely eyes. Among my Top 10 Beauty Foods, you'll find vitamin E in walnuts, blueberries, kiwifruit, spinach, and tomatoes. Other foods rich in vitamin E include peaches, prunes, cabbage, asparagus, avocados, and nuts and seeds. (For more information, see Chapter 3.)

- **Increase your intake of beta-carotene**, which has antioxidant effects and which the body converts into vitamin A, an important eye nutrient that helps the eye adapt from bright light to darkness. Among my Top 10 Beauty Foods, you'll find significant amounts of beta-carotene in sweet potatoes, spinach, kiwi, and tomatoes. You can also add beta-carotene to your diet with foods like pumpkin, carrots, chilies, mangoes, cantaloupe, and apricots. (For more information, see the sidebar at the end of this chapter.) Among my Top 10 Beauty Foods, good sources of retinol, the active form of vitamin A found in animal sources, are oysters, yogurt, and salmon. Other sources include milk, cheddar cheese, and eggs.

- **Consume foods rich in lutein and zeaxanthin**, the related carotenoids that are especially protective of your enchanting eyes. One recent study published in *Skin Pharmacology and Physiology* showed that lutein and zeaxanthin provide photoprotection when used topically, orally, or both—but the dietary approach shows the most promise. Specifically, the study concluded that oral administration of lutein may provide better protection than that afforded by topical application of this antioxidant when measured by changes in lipid peroxidation and photoprotective activity in the skin following UV light irradiation. Among my Top 10 Beauty Foods, lutein and zeaxanthin are found in spinach, blueberries, kiwifruit, and tomatoes. They are also found in egg yolks, as well as in green vegetables such as kale, turnip greens, collard greens, romaine lettuce, broccoli, zucchini, corn, garden peas, and Brussels sprouts. The lutein in egg yolks appears to be more bioavailable. Research has revealed that eating one egg a day significantly raises lutein and zeaxanthin levels.

- **Eat plenty of foods rich in zinc.** This mineral is essential to eye function, and its antioxidant effects protect the tissues of the eye from the damaging effects of UV light. Zinc also has countless other beauty benefits. Among my Top 10 Beauty Foods, oysters are a super source of zinc. You also can add more zinc to your diet with meats, seafood, liver, milk and other dairy products, beans, and whole grains. (For more information, see Chapter 3.)
- **Increase your intake of omega-3 fatty acids**, the super beauty food that supports healthy eyes. Choose cold-water fish like salmon, mackerel, herring, sardines, and trout. Add walnuts, spinach, flax, hemp seeds, pumpkin seeds, and soybeans to your diet (for more information, see Chapter 1).
- **Avoid sugar.** It has been known for a long time that the high blood sugar levels associated with diabetes harm the lens of the eye. Now scientists have determined that even if you don't have diabetes, you are putting your eyes at risk if you regularly consume carbohydrates that quickly raise your blood sugar level. A 2007 article in the *American Journal of Clinical Nutrition* concluded that a high-glycemic-index diet significantly increases the risk of age-related macular degeneration in people who do not have diabetes (see "Beauty Bite: Hidden Sugar" in Chapter 3).

Eating to Ease Dry Eye

It's hard to look fresh and dewy when your eyes feel like sandpaper! Nothing kills a glistening gaze like dry eye, a condition that affects millions, especially women. Symptoms include a feeling of dryness along with itching, irritation, blurred vision, sensitivity to light, and feeling like something is in your eye. Eyes can become dry either because you are not producing enough tears or because the tears you have are

BEAUTY MYTH

Eating Carrots Will Improve Your Eyesight

Are your eyeglasses cramping your style? Are you tired of searching for lost contact lenses? Go ahead and eat more carrots—but don't throw away your contacts or glasses. Including carrots in your diet won't keep you from needing glasses or correct your nearsightedness or farsightedness. Strictly speaking, carrots cannot improve your sight. However, the beta-carotene in carrots will help keep your eyes healthy because it is converted by the body into vitamin A, a vitamin that is especially protective of eye health. In your retinas, vitamin A helps prevent night blindness (the inability to see in the dark). Generally we think of beta-carotene as being converted into vitamin A in the liver, but it also is converted by the eye itself, by the retinal pigment epithelial cells. The presence of this alternative pathway suggests that the body does not want to take any chances when it comes to having a constant supply of vital vitamin A to protect your eyes.

evaporating at an unusually high rate. Common causes of dry eye include air-conditioning, forced-air heat, cigarette smoke, high altitude, prolonged use of the computer, long periods of driving, wearing contact lenses, and exposure to environmental factors like wind, dust, and allergens. Certain medications—including antihistamines, diuretics, oral contraceptives, and some antidepressants—can cause dry eye, and the condition also can be caused by aging, hormonal changes due to menopause, and different illnesses.

If you find yourself reaching regularly for a bottle of artificial tears to ease your eyes, make an appointment with an eye doctor before the problem progresses. Dry eye may become so severe that reading, driving, working, and other activities become difficult or impossible.

Beauty Nutrients Related to Dry Eye

Vitamin A deficiency can cause dry eye. The typical American diet has adequate amounts of vitamin A, but you may

BEAUTY MYTH

If You Get a Black Eye, Put a Steak on It

According to this old wives' tale, "enzymes" in the steak will help a black eye heal. Is there any truth to this advice?

No scientific evidence supports using a raw steak to heal a black eye. Using raw meat may actually cause more harm than good, since it contains potentially dangerous bacteria that could do serious harm, especially on sensitive areas such as the eye.

What a raw steak has going for it is temperature. The meat is cold, and that is what reduces swelling—not any extraordinary therapeutic enzymes or other magical properties of raw steak. Your best bet is to use an ice pack, a cold compress, or even a bag of frozen vegetables (wrapped in a clean cloth) during the first 24 hours to minimize bruising and swelling.

have problems absorbing nutrients from the foods you eat, or you may not be eating enough foods that contain either retinol or beta-carotene. Boosting your consumption of whole, natural foods rich in retinol or beta-carotene will provide your body with plenty of beauty-enhancing vitamin A. Many people take vitamin A supplements, but when it is taken in large amounts, vitamin A can accumulate in the body to toxic levels.

If your dry eyes are accompanied by dry skin and brittle nails, you may not be getting enough omega-3 fatty acids, which help keep your skin hydrated. A study published in the *American Journal of Clinical Nutrition* found that a high intake of omega-3 fatty acids protects against dry eye. In the study, women with the highest levels of omega-3 fats in their diets reduced their risk of dry eye syndrome by 20 percent compared to women with the lowest levels of these fats in their diet. Additionally, women who reported eating at least five servings of tuna per week had a 68 percent reduced risk of dry eye, compared to women who ate only one serving of tuna per week. A higher intake of omega-6 fatty acids, found in many cooking and salad oils and animal meats, may increase the risk of dry eye syndrome.

Bags Begone: The Diet to Defeat Dark Circles

The night before a photo shoot, celebrities are typically on their best behavior because nothing affects your face like last night's party. Puffiness around your eyes can send a variety of messages, from "I had the greatest night of my life last night!" to "I was just crying in the bathroom; leave me alone."

Puffy eyes can be caused by fluid retention due to a high salt intake or common problems like sleep deprivation, allergies, and nasal congestion. They also can be associated with more serious health problems, such as high blood pressure, congestive heart failure, liver disease, and kidney problems. Women are at added risk for water retention the week before menstruation. Estrogen replacement therapy and the birth control pill also can make your body retain water.

Dark circles under the eyes are unique to each individual. Many people come by them honestly—that is, they inherited them! Pale, translucent skin can make the bluish veins under the eye more apparent, making the area look darker. Sometimes this is part of the natural aging process, but sometimes people are pale because they didn't get enough sleep or they have health problems like anemia. Dark circles under the eyes can also be caused by dehydration, sudden weight loss, and smoking.

When you follow my Beauty Diet, you will boost circulation to your skin and avoid any diet-induced puffiness. People will notice your clear, sparkling eyes—not the bags beneath them!

THE BEAUTY DIET RX

For Clear, Refreshed Eyes

If your face looks a little puffy due to water retention, here are some changes you can make in your diet that might help:

- **Drink plenty of water.** Limiting liquid will not prevent water retention. Providing lots of water encourages the body to release it.

- **Enjoy green tea.** This beauty beverage is a source of caffeine, which acts as a diuretic.

- **Avoid foods high in sodium.** A high-salt diet raises the level of sodium in your blood and body fluids. In this environment, cells hold on to extra water and enlarge. Foods high in sodium include:

  1. ¼ cup miso soup: 2,516 mg

  2. 1 teaspoon table salt: 2,346 mg

  3. 1 can anchovies: 1,651 mg

  4. 1 tablespoon soy sauce: 1,029 mg

  5. 1 medium dill pickle: 833 mg

  6. ½ cup canned tomato sauce: 738 mg

  7. 1 tablespoon teriyaki sauce: 690 mg

  8. 1 ounce cured salt pork: 404 mg

  9. Processed foods, fast foods, and canned soups: quantity varies

- **Get enough B vitamins.** They may be effective in reducing water retention. The various B vitamins work together in the body, so eat a wide variety of foods to be sure you get all of them. Among my Top 10 Beauty Foods, the best source of thiamin (B_1) and biotin (B_7) is walnuts, the best source of riboflavin (B_2) and pantothenic acid (B_5) is yogurt, the best source of niacin (B_3) is wild salmon, the best source of folate (B_9) is spinach, and the best source of cobalamin (B_{12})—which is available only from animal sources—is oysters. Spinach, walnuts, and salmon are all good sources of pyridoxine (B_6).

How to Keep Your Eyes Wide— or Fake It

Here are some tips and tricks for looking bright-eyed and alert—even when you're feeling the opposite!

- Most people have puffy eyes in the morning. Usually the puffiness clears up as you stand up and go about your day. If you seriously don't want to wake up with puffy eyes, try sleeping on pillows that keep your head elevated.
- To help eliminate dark circles under your eyes, get more beauty sleep.
- To avoid wrinkles, don't spend extended periods of time in front of a computer or television screen. Avoid any activity that stresses the eyes and causes you to squint. To diminish an existing line, you can try sleeping with a piece of tape over it.
- Wear sunglasses. Bright sunlight makes you squint and contributes to wrinkles; plus, the UV light harms both your eyes and the delicate skin around your eyes.
- Relax. Finding ways to relax not only can reduce dark circles but also is incredibly beneficial to your overall appearance (see Chapter 8).
- Apply soothing substances to your eyes, including green tea, chamomile, cucumber, witch hazel, ginkgo, and aloe vera. For a home remedy, soak chamomile tea bags in ice water until they're really cold, squeeze out the water, then place the bags on your eyelids for 15 to 20 minutes. An alternative is to use cold cucumber slices or simply a cold cloth. Both the cool compresses and the relaxation will help your appearance.
- Shape your brows so they have an arch that opens the area above your eyes. However, don't try to redraw the brows nature gave you.
- Use an under-eye moisturizer specifically designed for the area. Some contain skin lighteners, while others are

supposed to shrink capillaries. Keeping skin moist will diminish wrinkles.

- Line your eyes, but to make them appear larger, don't line them all the way around with the same color. Try a darker shade on top and a lighter shade below.

Expert Advice: Makeup Tips for Beautiful Eyes

My friend Giella produces her own custom-blended cosmetics for the high-end department store Henri Bendel in New York City. I asked Giella for her expert advice for using makeup to enhance your eyes, especially when it comes to getting rid of dark circles and bags. Here's what she had to say:

Concealing dark circles is always a challenge. Here are some rules: Light colors give a more pronounced look, and dark colors recede. It's important to get the perfect combination of light and dark colors to disguise dark circles. Typically, concealers are too light, and that just makes circles more apparent. One tip is to blend two colors: one color that has a peach tone to cancel the skin's blue and another that is lighter to brighten the eye.

When blending, always use a concealer brush. It makes it much easier to control the coverage. A synthetic brush, made out of Taklon, has the feel of silk but the firmness of synthetic hairs. A brush will also warm up the concealer when stroking it, making it easier to apply. You can paint it on very lightly by using the tip of your brush, or you can use the flat side of the brush for a larger area. Remember, put concealer only where you need it. For example, you may not need it completely under your eyes. Typically, the inner corner of your eyes is sufficient. After applying the concealer with your brush, tap it with your ring finger (tap, tap, tap) until it disappears. Do not rub.

Vitamin A's Role in Beauty

Recommended Dietary Allowance

WOMEN	MEN
700 RE (2,333 IU)	900 RE (3,000 IU)

Vitamin A is a natural skin smoother. It is also important to healthy bones, teeth, hair, and fingernails. The active form of vitamin A (retinyl palmitate, a storage form of retinol) is found only in animal food sources. However, the precursor of vitamin A is beta-carotene, a plant compound with antioxidant properties. Your body can convert beta-carotene into vitamin A. While it is possible to take too many vitamin A supplements (do not exceed 10,000 IU per day, and exercise caution if you are simultaneously using a vitamin A–based medication, especially if you are considering pregnancy), it is not possible to overdose on beta-carotene.

Five Good Whole-Food Sources of Vitamin A

1. Beef liver, 3 oz.	9,196 RE
2. Chicken liver, 3 oz.	4,211 RE
3. Cheddar cheese, 1 oz.	86 RE
4. Egg, 1 boiled	84 RE
5. Swiss cheese, 1 oz.	65 RE

Five Good Whole-Food Sources of Beta-Carotene (Which the Body Can Convert to Vitamin A)

1. Pumpkin, canned, 1 cup	5,382 RE
2. Sweet potato, baked with skin, 1	2,487 RE
3. Carrot, raw, 1 medium	2,025 RE
4. Mango, 1 medium	805 RE
5. Spinach, boiled, ½ cup	737 RE

RE = retinol equivalents

Skin texture can make bags or circles look more pronounced. If skin is dry and dehydrated, eyes look much older, so keep the area concealed and hydrated. Use nourishing oils with anti-inflammatory properties to condition skin:

- Grapeseed oil is an excellent healing oil that contains linoleic acid, an essential fatty acid. It is a pale green moisturizer that is lighter and more absorbent than most oils. It is a good choice for those with nut allergies.
- Another good oil to try is emu oil, a natural oil with anti-inflammatory and moisturizing properties. The product is obtained from the fat of emu birds from Australia. Emu oil also contains essential fatty acids.
- Kukui oil comes from the candlenut tree. This rare Hawaiian plant oil is high in essential fatty acids for the maintenance of healthy skin. It is light and nongreasy and easily absorbed by the skin.
- Avocado oil lubricates and nourishes the skin and is a rich source of vitamin E. Avocado oil has the highest penetration rate of any plant oil, making it an excellent base for skin preparations. It also is antibacterial.
- Soybean oil has long been used in cooking, but lately this oil has grown in popularity for its use in cosmetic applications such as soap, body butter, lip and body balms, face creams and lotions, etc.
- Soy butter is another delicious addition for the skin. You can use it alone or mix it in with your concealer. It is a soft material that spreads easily on the skin, making it easier for concealer to glide on.

If your eyes are prone to puffiness, try keeping your concealer and/or creams in the refrigerator. Coolness helps reduce inflammation.

A new lightening powder on the market comes from *Phyllanthus emblica,* or the Indian gooseberry. It is mostly helpful when dealing with hyperpigmentation. It can be added to eye cream or concealer to actually lighten dark circles. Significant lightening has been seen after 8 to 10 weeks of use.

The Beauty Diet Lifestyle

Fitness—if it came in a bottle,
everybody would have a great body.
    —*Cher*

S o far I've shared my best advice for keeping your skin clear and smooth; maintaining your full, luxuriant, shiny hair; nurturing your long, strong, shapely fingernails; protecting your healthy, gleaming smile; and nourishing your bright, sparkling eyes. I've drawn on the latest scientific studies and offered you proven recommendations for enhancing your natural beauty from head to toe. I've provided you with vital information about nutrition, and in the chapter after this one I'll give you specific meal plans that offer an abundance of savory snacks and mouthwatering meals that all make use of my Top 10 Beauty Foods. If you read this book from beginning to end and follow my Beauty Diet, you will begin to see wonderful changes in your appearance from the inside out, in as little as four weeks.

But adopting nutritional habits that enhance your health and beauty is only one part of the journey. The Beauty Diet would not be complete without mentioning some other aspects of daily life that play an important role in how you look and feel. I'm talking about your willingness to physically challenge your body and your ability to decompress from the various stressors that surround you. So, in addition to telling you about the best foods and nutrients to consume for optimal beauty, I feel it is pertinent to tell you about lifestyle factors that affect your appearance, including physical activities and behaviors that encourage and maintain your attractiveness and health. Here are the best beauty-enhancing lifestyle secrets I've found—and used myself!

Staying Fit and Fabulous

As a woman concerned with beauty, you're probably pretty finely attuned to the changes you've seen in your body over the past few years. Maybe your body has adjusted to adult life with a little more sagging—a body your partner describes as "cushy." Maybe you've acquired some dreaded cellulite in areas you never could have imagined. And if these are unhappy thoughts, let your mind wander for a bit to the changes you can't see—changes that impact your overall health. To get the whole package—a boost in confidence, a higher energy level, antiaging benefits, and an all-around healthier and more beautiful body—you absolutely must add exercise to the mix.

The Beauty and Health Benefits of Exercise

In addition to offering various health benefits, exercise improves your posture, balance, and coordination. Being graceful is an important part of being attractive! Exercise also burns calories, helping you stay slim and beautiful (see "Burning Calories with Exercise"). Bodies require a certain amount of energy to sustain life, but once you've fulfilled that need, the rest is just excess calories that get stored as fat, unless you burn them off. Weight-bearing exercise is particularly important because it builds muscle, and since muscle is the most metabolically active tissue in the body, the more muscle you have, the more calories you'll burn—even when you are sitting. By helping you stay slim, exercise not only keeps you looking fantastic but also fights obesity and all the health problems associated with it, including heart disease, diabetes, and cancer.

A healthier and more beautiful body is just one dimension of the benefits of exercise. A whole other dimension lies with your state of mind. Exercise can lift your mood and is a great way to manage stress. Research has shown that exercise elevates levels of serotonin (a brain chemical responsible for feelings of calmness and relaxation) to provide an instant lift. Just 30 minutes of moderate to vigorous aerobic exercise—done at 60 to 75 percent of your maximum heart rate—has been shown to significantly improve both mood and energy levels. Exercise also stimulates endorphins, other neurotransmitters that provide natural pain relief and make you feel good all over.

Burning Calories with Exercise

The number of calories you burn during different activities depends on several factors, including your weight and how long and vigorously you exercise. Following are some figures for someone who weighs 150 pounds and spends 20 minutes on various activities. Note: these numbers should be used as rough estimates because technique can vary widely.

Bicycling (moderate effort)	191
Bicycling (stationary bike, vigorous effort)	250

Bowling	71
Boxing (punching a heavy bag)	143
Carrying groceries upstairs	179
Dancing (disco)	107
Dancing (ballroom, waltz)	71
Dancing (modern, jazz, tap, ballet)	114
Gardening	95
Jumping rope, fast	286
Kayaking	119
Roller-blading	286
Running (5 mph)	191
Scrubbing the floor (on hands and knees)	90
Sexual activity	31
Shoveling snow	143
Skiing (downhill)	119
Skiing (cross-country, moderate speed)	191
Stair treadmill	214
Swimming (laps, fast, vigorous effort)	238
Swimming (laps, moderate effort)	167
Tennis (singles)	191
Vacuuming	83
Walking (moderate pace, 3 mph)	79
Walking (very brisk pace, 4 mph)	119
Yoga (stretching)	60

Data calculated on bodybuilding.com.

Finding the Fun in Fitness

Exercise doesn't have to mean endless hours of pain and boredom. In fact, it can be fun! It's *your* workout, so your job is to personalize it just as you would your home décor or your wedding. Following are some forms of exercise that I feel best promote beauty *and* satisfy the desire to have fun.

BEAUTY MYTH

Weight Training Gives Women Big, Bulky Muscles

Some women are afraid of weight training because they don't want to get big, bulky muscles. I, for one, can attest that I used to avoid weights out of fear of getting too bulky. But after doing some research, I discovered this is a myth: strength training does not make you look like a bodybuilder unless you *want* to look like a bodybuilder. Women ordinarily do not have enough testosterone to create giant muscles. Working out with weights, stretch bands, or resistance tubing is extremely beneficial to women because we naturally have less muscle and bone than men, and we begin to lose both with age. So, it is one of the best things we can do to counteract these inevitable changes. Overall, strength training is a terrific way to look beautiful and toned while relieving stress. After overcoming my fear of weights, I can tell you my arms looked great in my wedding dress!

Dancing up a Storm

There are so many kinds of dancing that one of them is sure to suit you. Bellydancing? Irish dancing? Modern dance? Ballet? Jazz? Ballroom dancing has become increasingly popular with my favorite TV show "Dancing with the Stars"!

Wherever there's music, there's dancing. Take your dancing up a notch and you'll burn calories, tone your muscles, improve your circulation, and boost your mood and energy level. Dancing can increase your strength, endurance, and flexibility, plus it relieves stress and lets you be creative.

Dancing can be as convenient and affordable as you want it to be. You can sign up for private ballroom dance lessons (I take lessons with my husband, David) or just put on your favorite CD and boogie.

You'll get cardiovascular benefits from dancing three times a week for 20 minutes. If you goal is to lose weight, you'll need to stay on your toes a little longer. There are many different ways to dance your way to fitness, so to make it fun, pick more than one.

Mindful Exercise: Yoga and Tai Chi

Over the past 10 years, yoga and tai chi have established their own growing sector of the fitness world called *mindful exercise*. These forms of exercise are so wildly popular that they're often on the daily schedules at fitness centers. The reason so many women can be seen sporting their own yoga mats and shoulder bags on any given Saturday is that these are exercises that work your body while relaxing your mind.

Yoga is no passing trend. In fact, it's more than 5,000 years old. Because of its gentle nature, yoga is suitable for most adults of any age or fitness level. When it's practiced regularly, practitioners notice physical, emotional, and perhaps even spiritual effects of yoga.

If you're exploring the world of yoga, you should know that there is not just one type. There are actually many different practices of yoga, each focusing on a different set of benefits. Hatha yoga, the most popular form practiced in Western countries, focuses on breathing and posture. Other forms of yoga may focus on goals such as relaxation, intuition, or healing. But whatever the form, three integral tenets of yoga—exercise, breathing, and meditation—help students achieve their goals. To find out which form is right for you, head straight to your nearest yoga studio and try it out.

If you're a beginner, it's a good idea to take an introductory workshop. You may prefer to learn what downward dog looks like first, before hearing about it in class! I took an introductory workshop at my neighborhood favorite, New York Yoga, and it offered me an opportunity to learn various poses while receiving constructive feedback.

Tai chi is suitable for anyone who wants to move with greater strength, grace, and ease, from adolescents to the aged. This ancient Chinese method of movement is nonimpact. It incorporates flowing movements while shifting the body's balance.

Tai chi movements are performed slowly, evenly, and mindfully. The Chinese compare the movement to pulling the silk from a cocoon: pull steadily and the strand will unravel; pull too fast or too slow, and it breaks. In tai chi, the body is always moving, but under complete control as it remains soft and relaxed. Practiced for just 20 minutes a day, tai chi can relieve stress, increase flexibility, build stamina, and strengthen the body, all without any huffing and puffing on your part.

Pilates

People often ask me how I stay in such good shape, and I am happy to tell them, "Pilates!" Pilates exercises have been sculpting dancers' bodies for years. The method was developed in the early 1900s by German-born boxer and fitness enthusiast Joseph Pilates. He devised a series of physical movements that—coupled with focused breathing patterns—stretch, strengthen, and balance the body. He also invented unique equipment that challenges and supports the body during special exercises. The Pilates system is made up of a sequence of exercises meant to be followed in a certain order. The routines done on the floor are known as *matwork*, and they are complemented by the exercises that use equipment. In Pilates, exercises are done with careful precision and with only a few repetitions, maximizing the effects of the work by how the exercises are executed, not by the number of repetitions.

The first thing a Pilates instructor will tell you is that Pilates is not just a series of exercises but an approach to developing body awareness. The Pilates method has been described as an intelligent form of exercise—a holistic approach to the mind, body, and spirit that offers multiple benefits.

My Pilates instructor, Tara Bridger, told me during my first session that Pilates focuses on the body's core or "powerhouse"—the deep abdominals, lower back muscles, hips, and buttocks—and then extends outward to the rest of the body, providing balance, strength, posture, and efficient movement. It builds strength upward along the spine while supporting the other joints and muscles. Specific attention is also paid to strengthening the upper back muscles that draw the shoulders down and open the chest. When the exercises are done with precision and mental focus, you learn to feel your imbalances and to see how your body has compensated for them over the years. Tara explained to me that Pilates corrects these weaknesses, optimizes how the body functions, and teaches the body to remember its natural alignment and to move in the safest and most energy-efficient way. The overall benefits include a strong, flexible spine, deep core strength, increased muscle tone, greater flexibility, better alignment, stronger mental focus, increased circulation, decreased stress, greater energy, and, the benefit I have noticed the most during my sessions, improved posture. When correct posture is relearned (we all started with it, according to Tara), our presence becomes stronger and more attractive and we appear and eventually feel more confident.

Pilates creates a flat, strong tummy and builds long, lean muscles without bulk. How? Because the system was designed to lengthen and stretch the muscles as it strengthens them. Pilates has narrowed my waistline and toned my buttocks and thighs. It has defined the muscles in and around my spine and along my arms. Overall, it makes the whole body look and feel strong, supple, vibrant, and naturally beautiful. Tara tells me there are over 500 exercises in the Pilates system (I haven't learned them all yet!). Though every regimen strengthens the core and tones the whole body, the system allows for specific focus on whatever area of the body needs the most attention, because every body is different.

Expert Advice: Finding the Right Pilates Instructor

I asked Tara Bridger for her insights about finding a Pilates teacher. Tara is a certified Pilates instructor and an expert in the method taught by Romana Kryzanowska, a protégé of Joseph Pilates. This is what she had to say:

Because the title *Pilates* can be used to describe any type of exercise that incorporates some aspect of the original Pilates method, you'll want to take the time to find a legitimate, effective, and safe studio with reputable instructors.

The original method designed and taught by Joseph Pilates is practiced today at studios that trained under the Romana's Pilates Method or Authentic Pilates Method. Joseph Pilates chose Romana Kryzanowska to carry on his legacy before he died in 1967. Today Romana is in her 80s and still teaching throughout the country. She continues to be the foundation of his method. It's taught by instructors who either trained directly under Romana or under one of her direct Pilates descendants. Many branches of Pilates have altered or diffused the original system and have implemented new exercises and techniques that are not technically Pilates. The original method and its followers subscribe to a very high standard of practice.

On a more personal level, you want to find an atmosphere you feel comfortable in and an instructor whose personality and approach work best with you. Do you prefer a private setting where no other clients are present? Or are you more comfortable when others are exercising around you? Some studios are larger and can accommodate many private sessions at once, while others offer a more spalike environment. Do you prefer a man or a woman? A softer, gentler, encouraging voice? Or someone with a tougher "coach" quality who is ready to push you when you need it? Finding the best instructor for you is a trial-and-error process. I recommend trying a few different people at first. Also, it may be beneficial to work with more than one person on an ongoing basis to gain different perspectives. Everyone has a different eye, even though all should be teaching the same technique. You'll know when you're with the right person. Trust your instincts!

Look beyond just the mat classes. Understand that to fully benefit from Pilates you should practice the entire system, which involves the equipment (Reformer, Cadillac, Wunda Chair, etc.) as well as the mat. Be wary of studios that offer group classes on the equipment, especially the Reformer. Pilates cannot be taught safely on the Reformer in groups of more than three people. A larger class size means the system has been greatly modified from its original form to be taught in groups.

It is important to have some one-on-one instruction and experience with the whole system before diving into a large class setting—both for safety reasons and for the effectiveness of the workout. Large classes combine people with different levels of strength and various body types and limitations. If you are not in a financial position to take private lessons on an ongoing basis, either invest in a series of 5 to 10 private sessions and then proceed into classes (and brush up with a private lesson about once a month), or look into duets or trios, which still offer individual attention for considerably less money.

Be sure your instructor follows strict safety guidelines. The Pilates system should always be taught by an instructor who adheres to the "safety first" policy. If the equipment is misused or a client is worked beyond his or her strength level, injuries can occur.

If you have concerns about whether or not a studio or instructor is appropriate, you can always contact the two studios in New York that train instructors under the original Pilates method: True Pilates (212-757-0724) or the New York

Pilates Studio (212-245-8367) to see what affiliations they have in your city.

For Inner and Outer Beauty: Stress Less

A life filled with beauty from the inside out begins with eating healthfully, including my Top 10 Beauty Foods in your diet, and adding exercise to your daily routine. There's just one more part of your life that needs attention. You'll also need to decrease your stress—an inevitable factor in life that detracts from your beautiful appearance and ruins your calm demeanor. In addition to exercise, R & R (rest and relaxation) are key to looking and feeling your best. The more relaxed you are, the better you feel and the more beautiful you look.

Tension Is the Enemy of Beauty

We all know that stress exacerbates skin conditions like acne and that being constantly tired and worried makes people look old. But for many years there was no scientific explanation for this mind/body connection. When a 2004 study published in the *Proceedings of the National Academy of Sciences* showed a connection between life stress and looking old, this seemed like a blinding flash of the obvious, but it was a big deal in scientific circles. The study compared biological markers between a group of women who cared for a chronically ill child and a control group of women with healthy children. The study found that the more years of caregiving a woman had experienced, the shorter the length of her telomeres (the caps of DNA protein on chromosomes that are reduced every time a cell divides), the lower her telomerase activity (an enzyme that protects telomeres), and the greater her oxidative stress. Additionally, the telomeres of women with the highest *perceived* psychological stress—across both groups—had undergone the equivalent of approximately 10 years of additional aging, compared with the women across both groups who had the lowest perception of being stressed.

Stress can contribute to wrinkles and may aggravate skin conditions including eczema and acne. The effects of stress not only can show up in your face, but also around your middle! If you've ever gone through half a bag of Hershey's Kisses without realizing it, you know there is a link between anxiety and eating.

Adding Relaxing Moments to Your Life

Busy lives don't lend themselves to long periods of relaxation on a daily, weekly, or even monthly basis. But the key is not the length of time you incorporate relaxation into your daily life. The most important thing is that you make some time for it, even if it's very small, on a regular basis.

Anything that allows your mind to escape the stresses of life can be helpful in making you feel calm and at peace. In addition to dancing and Pilates, here are some of my favorite stress-reducing activities.

CREATE A RELAXATION ROOM AT HOME. Many spas have relaxation rooms to sit in before and after treatments. It's great to create a relaxation space at home too. It doesn't have to be a "room" per se—it can be a space in your bedroom, for example—but the key is having an area at home that is devoted solely to relaxing. You may want to add a really comfortable chair or daybed, put a dimmer on the lights, or have candles on hand—whatever it is that you enjoy and find relaxing. This will give you an opportunity to decompress. The key is not to have too many outside stimuli. Forget the BlackBerry, cell phone, and laptop; this is a time to unwind and clear your mind of distractions and stressors.

MEDITATE. Meditation is a great way to relax, especially if you are under a lot of stress. Research has shown that meditation can lower heart rate and blood pressure and even improve cognitive performance. Important factors to consider when meditating include finding a comfortable place, relaxing your muscles, and focusing on one thing, whether it's your breathing, an object (a flower or a painting), or even a picture in your mind. You might visualize a peaceful place, like a secret garden. Or you might imagine sitting on a beach in the Caribbean or standing on the summit of a mountain. Meditating for as little as 10 minutes is enough to have a beneficial effect on your stress level. The key is staying focused and not letting any distractions or thoughts enter your mind. This may be difficult at first and may take a lot of time and practice. Being mindful is key.

LISTEN TO YOUR FAVORITE MUSIC. Listening to soothing music can be very relaxing—and slow tempos in particular can induce a calm state of mind. Calming music can slow your breathing and heart rate, lower your blood pressure, and relax tense muscles too. This can be particularly beneficial when you're getting ready for a tough day at work, if you're in your car stuck in traffic, or if you're lying in bed trying to free your mind of stressful thoughts. Music therapy has been shown to be helpful in decreasing anxiety associated with medical procedures: one recent study from Temple University found that individuals who listened to music during a colonoscopy required less sedation during the procedure than those who didn't listen to their favorite tunes.

GET A MASSAGE. Having a massage is a great way to free yourself of tension, and adding aromatherapy oils such as chamomile or lavender can be particularly beneficial. One recent study found that emergency-room nurses experienced reduced stress levels with aromatherapy massage. The study, published in the *Journal of Clinical Nursing,* found that at least 50 percent of the emergency-room staff suffered moderate to extreme anxiety. However, this figure fell to 8 percent once staff received 15-minute aromatherapy massages while listening to music. While it may be preferable, you don't necessarily need a full hour to experience benefits!

TAKE A HOT BATH. Heat relaxes muscles—and taking a long bath can be soothing to the mind as well. Stock up on your favorite bath salts and soaps, get a bath pillow, and decorate the room with candles. You can even create an in-home spa by incorporating treatments like facials into your routine.

TAKE A VACATION. Even when you have a day off, it's hard to relax if you're surrounded by all the usual stressors—piles of bills, home repair jobs that need to be done, shopping to do, and all the other obligations of daily life that make your "to do" list go on for two pages. To escape your day-to-day worries, you need to escape your surroundings! For most people, a vacation to a warm climate, preferably on a sandy beach, is ideal. On the other hand, you may have always wanted to go to Alaska. Whether you prefer a no-frills campout or a luxury hotel, do whatever you find rejuvenating. If you can possibly swing it, get away to relax.

Getting Your Beauty Sleep

There's a reason they call it beauty sleep! A full, deep, restful sleep can help you stay healthy, lose weight, be more alert, improve your concentration, increase your productivity, elevate your mood—and ensure that you wake up gorgeous. You might be aware that you look and feel better after you get a good night's sleep!

Sleep is a time for your body to repair damage caused by everyday wear and tear as well as by sun exposure, stress, illness, and so on. During sleep the body focuses on regenerating cells and on maintaining and building bones, muscles, and other tissues. This kind of repair work also can occur while you're awake, but sleep allows the body to concentrate on healing without having to divide its energy sixteen different ways. While you are sleeping, you also recharge your immune system and rebalance the chemicals in your brain. In addition, you subconsciously process the day's events and even mull over problems—sometimes even producing bright ideas in the middle of the night. When you have a problem, it always helps to "sleep on it."

Sleep Yourself Thin

Researchers have uncovered an interesting connection between sleep and weight. People who do not get enough sleep are at increased risk of eating too much—not because they lack willpower, but because their hormones are working against them. Have you ever had a sleepless night, followed by a day when you just wanted to keep nibbling? Welcome to the effects of the hormones leptin and ghrelin.

Leptin and ghrelin work together to control feelings of hunger. Ghrelin is produced in the gastrointestinal tract and stimulates appetite. Leptin is produced by fat cells and sends a signal to the brain that you are full. Research shows that when you don't get enough sleep, it reduces your levels of leptin, so you don't feel as satisfied after you eat. Sleep loss also causes your levels of ghrelin to rise, which stimulates your appetite. This dynamic creates the perfect conditions for overeating. In fact, researchers have found that people who sleep less than seven hours per night are more likely to be overweight.

Two studies—the first conducted at the University of Chicago in Illinois and the second at Stanford University in California—reveal a great deal about how leptin and ghrelin operate. In the Chicago study, researchers subjected 12 healthy men in their 20s to two days of sleep deprivation, followed by two nights with 10 hours of sleep. During this time doctors monitored their hormone levels, appetite, and activity. After two nights of sleep deprivation, the participants' levels of leptin (the appetite suppressor) went down, and their levels of ghrelin (the appetite stimulator) went up. They experienced greater appetite, and they specifically craved high-sugar, high-salt, and starchy foods. The researchers were surprised to discover that hormone levels could be affected so much, in such a brief amount of time.

In the Stanford study, about 1,000 volunteers reported the number of hours they slept each night. Researchers tracked their levels of ghrelin and leptin and charted their weight. This study revealed that those who slept less than eight hours a night not only had lower levels of leptin and higher levels of ghrelin but also had a higher level of body fat. Specifically, there was 4 percent increase in body mass index when sleep was decreased from eight hours to five hours—a finding that can represent a difference of 25 pounds!

Conquering Insomnia

Waking up with a puffy face and bags under your eyes is an unfortunate consequence of insomnia. If you are having some problems getting your beauty sleep, here are some things to try:

- **Take a hot shower.** If you take a relaxing shower, then lie quietly in bed, it may be just what your body needs to get to sleep. If you have time, a hot bath—complete with scented candles and bath salts—is even more relaxing.
- **Open the window.** Fresh air and a cool room temperature provide the best sleeping conditions. If you need more warmth, buy a cozy comforter, but leave the air temperature cool.
- **Get comfortable.** The kind of mattress and pillow you like best will help you get comfortable right away. Few things are more annoying than trying to sleep in an old, worn-out mattress with a lousy pillow.
- **Write down your worries before bed.** Try to empty your brain of concerns by writing everything down before you turn out

the light. If you have any solutions or bright ideas, write them down too. This way you don't have to keep reminding yourself to remember something.

- **Keep to a sleep schedule.** Your body will respond to a regular routine. Your head may complain, but your body will thank you for going to bed and waking up at the same time every day—even on weekends.
- **Close the curtains.** Your eyes know what time of day it is and send a daytime/nighttime message directly to the pineal gland inside your brain. When your eyes sense darkness, your pineal gland produces melatonin and you get sleepy. On the other hand, when it's light, your body knows it's time for action. This is why, if you pull an all-nighter, you'll get a "second wind" at dawn the next morning even if you never get to sleep. Be sure your bedroom is dark to help your body produce the melatonin it needs.
- **Hide your clock.** A big, illuminated clock may make you feel stressed and anxious about the time that is passing while you toss and turn. Cover the face of your clock so you don't obsess about the time.
- **Cut out caffeine.** For some people, even a small amount of caffeine early in the day can cause problems with falling asleep 12 hours later. If you're sensitive to caffeine, stay away from coffee, caffeinated tea, chocolate, and soft drinks. If you aren't sure whether caffeine is a problem for you, try eliminating caffeinated food and beverages for one week and see if your sleeping patterns improve.
- **Avoid alcohol.** A glass of wine may make it easier to fall asleep, but drinking before bedtime increases the likelihood that you will wake up during the night. If you enjoy a drink at night, it's probably best to limit yourself to one alcoholic beverage with dinner.
- **Eat dinner early.** Too much food before bed can cause distention and discomfort, making it difficult to fall asleep or stay asleep. Also, fat takes longer to digest and may cause distention at night. Lying down makes heartburn worse, and

heartburn itself makes falling asleep more difficult. Heartburn also awakens sleepers with middle-of-the-night discomfort. Avoid large dinner meals and wait at least two hours after eating before going to sleep.

- **Avoid spicy foods.** Spicy foods can contribute to heartburn, which can make it difficult to fall asleep by causing discomfort throughout the night. Watch out for chilies, curry powder, and other offenders.

- **Exercise early.** Exercising right before going to bed can make falling asleep more difficult, as it wakes up your system, revs up your body temperature and metabolism, and can lead to increased alertness. It is best to complete your workout at least a few hours before bedtime. In general, exercising regularly makes it easier to fall asleep and contributes to sounder sleep. However, exercising sporadically or right before going to bed will make falling asleep more difficult. Late-afternoon exercise is the perfect way to help you fall asleep at night.

- **Don't smoke.** According to the National Sleep Foundation, new evidence suggests that smoking may negatively impact sleep. Researchers from Johns Hopkins University compared the EEG recordings of a group of cigarette smokers with those of a group of nonsmokers. They found that smokers spend less time in deep sleep, especially in the earlier part of the night, and they are more likely to report feeling unrefreshed after sleeping. Nicotine in tobacco products is a stimulant and contributes to sleep problems.

- **Have a small bedtime snack.** A glass of warm milk 15 minutes before going to bed will soothe your nervous system. Milk contains calcium, which works directly on jagged nerves to make them (and you) relax. You can also try a cup of hot tea. Most stores have special blends of herb tea designed to help you get to sleep.

- **Check to see if you have sleep apnea.** If you sense you aren't sleeping well, or if your partner notices you are snoring or waking up repeatedly because you can't breathe, go to a sleep clinic and find out if you have sleep apnea. This disorder interferes with your ability to get a good night's rest. Once it is corrected, you'll sleep better and have more energy—and many people report they are able to lose weight more easily.

Now that you are armed with my nutrition and lifestyle tips for feeling and looking fabulous, it's time to put it all into practice. To get started, turn the page to begin my delicious Beauty Diet!

The Beauty Diet Meal Plan

Welcome to the Beauty Diet! Each breakfast, lunch, dinner, and beauty snack on the four-week meal plan that follows contains at least one of my Top 10 Beauty Foods. By following the plan, you can maximize your intake of beauty nutrients while enjoying delicious recipes! I am confident you will savor the variety of flavors in the different meals and snacks, and the best part is you won't have to worry about your waistline because each day averages approximately 1,500 calories to help keep you slim. If you follow my Beauty Diet diligently, you can expect to see improvements in your appearance in about four short weeks.

The Beauty Diet menus form a four-week meal plan that you can follow on 28 consecutive days. Recipes for breakfasts, lunches, dinners, and snacks appear separately after the four weekly menus, and are listed alphabetically. You can feel free to mix and match the recipes within each week as you desire. As long as you use recipes from the same week, your weekly averages will reflect the nutritional analysis following each week's plan. After four weeks have passed, you can feel free to resume the Beauty Diet by starting again with week 1's meals and beauty snacks.

While I feel the menus provide you with the most flavorful and foolproof approach to consuming your daily quota of beauty nutrients, please keep in mind that you can use the Top 10 Beauty Foods to create your own meals and snacks. If you choose this more flexible approach, I recommend that you include at least one Top 10 Beauty Food in each of your three meals and two beauty snacks every day, and make sure that your daily calorie intake remains at approximately 1,500 calories.

Enjoy the Beauty Diet—and all of the glamorous beauty benefits that come with it!

The Beauty Diet Week 1 Menu (Days 1–7)

MONDAY
- **Breakfast:** Egg White, Spinach, and Feta Scramble on Whole Wheat Toast; 1 cup low-fat plain yogurt with ½ cup mixed berries
- **Lunch:** Lemon-Grilled Chicken over Mixed Green Salad with Yogurt Dill Dressing
- **Dinner:** Sautéed Mediterranean Shrimp, Tomatoes, and Broccoli over Whole Wheat Spaghetti
- **Beauty Snack 1:** 1 ounce Spiced Walnuts; one 8-ounce glass low-fat milk
- **Beauty Snack 2:** 1 ounce dark chocolate (60 percent cacao)

TUESDAY
- **Breakfast:** Triple-Berry Smoothie; 1 whole grain English muffin with 2 tablespoons peanut butter

- **Lunch:** Mango, Red Onion, Avocado, Spinach, and Crab Wrap; one 8-ounce glass low-fat milk
- **Dinner:** Herb-Baked Salmon with Warm Cherry Tomato Salad and Whole Wheat Couscous
- **Beauty Snack 1:** White Bean "Hummus" with five baby carrots and one kiwi
- **Beauty Snack 2:** Blueberry Yogurt Panna Cotta

WEDNESDAY

- **Breakfast:** French Toast Stuffed with Ricotta, Kiwi, and Peach
- **Lunch:** Sweet Potato Leek Soup; ½ whole wheat pita with 3 ounces sliced turkey, lettuce, tomato, and mustard
- **Dinner:** Grilled Halibut and Vegetable Skewers; 2 cups mesclun greens with 1 teaspoon extra virgin olive oil and 1 tablespoon balsamic vinegar
- **Beauty Snack 1:** Raspberry Almond Yogurt Cup
- **Beauty Snack 2:** Pomegranate Blueberry Smoothie

THURSDAY

- **Breakfast:** 2 slices whole wheat toast with 1 ounce light cream cheese and 2 slices tomato; one 8-ounce glass low-fat milk
- **Lunch:** Curry Chicken Salad over Baby Spinach; ¼ cup almonds
- **Dinner:** Poached Oysters in Garlic, Herbs, and Broth with Mixed Greens and Whole Wheat Baguette
- **Beauty Snack 1:** Nutty Banana Shake
- **Beauty Snack 2:** 1 cup mixed berries; 1 ounce dark chocolate (60 percent cacao)

FRIDAY

- **Breakfast:** Whole grain English muffin with 2 tablespoons peanut butter; one 8-ounce glass low-fat milk; ½ cup blueberries
- **Lunch:** Lobster Salad Sandwich with a Creamy Yogurt Dressing

- **Dinner:** Grilled Chicken Skewers with Yogurt Cucumber Sauce and Cherry Tomato Couscous
- **Beauty Snack 1:** Cranberry Orange Granita with Dark Chocolate Shavings
- **Beauty Snack 2:** Kiwi Melon Fruit Salad with Ginger Blueberry Syrup

SATURDAY

- **Breakfast:** Steel-Cut Oats Cooked with Milk, Berries, and Walnuts
- **Lunch:** Roast Beef, Arugula, and Tomato Wrap; one 4-ounce glass low-fat milk
- **Dinner:** Spiced Salmon with Roasted Broccoli
- **Beauty Snack 1:** Maple Yogurt Crunch
- **Beauty Snack 2:** Dark Chocolate Fondue with Strawberries; one 8-ounce glass low-fat milk

SUNDAY

- **Breakfast:** Scrambled Egg Whites with Cheddar and Tomato and Sliced Kiwi; one 8-ounce glass low-fat milk
- **Lunch:** Spicy Carrot and Sweet Potato Soup; multigrain roll
- **Dinner:** Lemony Roasted Chicken and Artichokes with Garlicky Wilted Spinach
- **Beauty Snack 1:** 1 ounce Parmesan cheese; 1 ounce Spiced Walnuts
- **Beauty Snack 2:** Black and Blue Yogurt Parfait

DAILY AVERAGE FOR WEEK 1

1,440 calories; 98 g protein; 160 g carbohydrates; 23 g fiber; 48 g fat; 12 g saturated fat; 0 trans fats; 189 mg cholesterol; 2,064 mg sodium; 1,006 mg calcium; 3 g omega-3 fats

The Beauty Diet Week 2 Menu (Days 8–14)

MONDAY
- **Breakfast:** 1 cup whole grain cereal, such as Kashi GoLean, with ½ cup blueberries and ½ cup low-fat milk
- **Lunch:** Anytime Thanksgiving Salad
- **Dinner:** Walnut-Crusted Salmon with Buttermilk Scallion Smashed Sweet Potatoes and Roasted Broccoli
- **Beauty Snack 1:** Vanilla Orange "Creamsicle" Smoothie
- **Beauty Snack 2:** Creamy Chocolate Cherry Rice Pudding

TUESDAY
- **Breakfast:** Strawberry Raspberry Yogurt Parfait
- **Lunch:** Hummus and Grilled Vegetable Wrap; 2 sliced kiwis
- **Dinner:** Asian Citrus Halibut with Brown Rice and Garlicky Wilted Spinach
- **Beauty Snack 1:** Blueberry Ginger Smoothie
- **Beauty Snack 2:** Dark Chocolate–Dipped Frozen Bananas

WEDNESDAY
- **Breakfast:** 2 pieces whole wheat toast with 1 ounce light cream cheese, 1 ounce smoked salmon, 2 slices tomato, and 2 tablespoons finely chopped red onion
- **Lunch:** Greek Tuna and Spinach Salad with Yogurt Dill Dressing
- **Dinner:** Braised Chicken with Dried Fruit over Toasted Walnut Couscous
- **Beauty Snack 1:** Raspberry Lemon Yogurt Cup
- **Beauty Snack 2:** 1 cup blueberries; 1 ounce Parmesan cheese

THURSDAY
- **Breakfast:** Banana Blueberry Yogurt Cup
- **Lunch:** Artichoke Bruschetta Salad
- **Dinner:** Garlic Herb Lobster Tail with Spinach and Pea Risotto

- **Beauty Snack 1:** 1 ounce dark chocolate (60 percent cacao); 1 cup mixed berries
- **Beauty Snack 2:** Tomato, Mozzarella, and Basil Stack

FRIDAY

- **Breakfast:** Scrambled Egg Whites with Cheddar and Tomato and Sliced Kiwi and 2 slices whole wheat toast
- **Lunch:** Roasted Vegetable Pita Pizza with Herbed Goat Cheese Medallions
- **Dinner:** Shrimp, Sweet Potato, and Vegetable Curry over Coconut-Lime Jasmine Rice
- **Beauty Snack 1:** Tropical Kiwi Fruit Salad with Vanilla Lime Syrup
- **Beauty Snack 2:** 1 ounce Spiced Walnuts; 1 8-ounce glass low-fat milk

SATURDAY

- **Breakfast:** Oatmeal with Cinnamon, Dried Fruit, and Toasted Walnuts
- **Lunch:** Lime- and Cilantro-Marinated Chicken with Roasted Corn, Black Bean, and Tomato Salad
- **Dinner:** Grilled Salmon with Mango Kiwi Salsa with Grilled Sweet Potato "Fries"
- **Beauty Snack 1:** Sweet and Spicy Yogurt
- **Beauty Snack 2:** Quick Mexican Hot Dark Chocolate

SUNDAY

- **Breakfast:** Tomato Scallion Frittata with Turkey Bacon
- **Lunch:** Ham, Zucchini, Red Onion, Spinach, and Ricotta Panini
- **Dinner:** Oysters on the Half Shell with Fresh Tomato Mignonette, Mixed Green Salad, and Whole Wheat Baguette
- **Beauty Snack 1:** Maple Yogurt Crunch
- **Beauty Snack 2:** Peach Blueberry Ginger Crisp; one 8-ounce glass low-fat milk

DAILY AVERAGE FOR WEEK 2

1,494 calories; 95 g protein; 175 g carbohydrates; 25 g
  fiber; 50 g fat; 15 g saturated fat; 0 trans fats; 218 mg
  cholesterol; 2,279 mg sodium; 1,021 mg calcium; 3 g
  omega-3 fats

The Beauty Diet Week 3 Menu (Days 15–21)

MONDAY

- **Breakfast:** Whole Grain Blueberry Pancakes; one 8-ounce glass low-fat milk
- **Lunch:** Grilled Chicken Sandwich with Walnut Basil Pesto and Fresh Mozzarella
- **Dinner:** Mustard-Crusted Salmon with Roasted Green Beans and Shallots
- **Beauty Snack 1:** Blackberry Yogurt
- **Beauty Snack 2:** Dark Chocolate–Dipped Pretzels

TUESDAY

- **Breakfast:** Poached Eggs Florentine; 1 cup mixed berries
- **Lunch:** Sweet and Spicy Crab and Kiwi Salad
- **Dinner:** Oven-Crunchy Walnut Chicken Tenders with Sweet Potato Hash
- **Beauty Snack 1:** Green Tea Frozen Yogurt
- **Beauty Snack 2:** 1 ounce Spiced Walnuts; one 8-ounce glass low-fat milk

WEDNESDAY

- **Breakfast:** 1 cup whole grain cereal, such as Kashi GoLean, with ½ cup blueberries and ½ cup low-fat milk
- **Lunch:** California Turkey Burger with Creamy Avocado Yogurt Spread

- **Dinner:** Shrimp and Angel Hair Pasta with Baby Spinach and Sliced Mushroom Salad
- **Beauty Snack 1:** Roasted Peaches with Walnut Crumb Filling
- **Beauty Snack 2:** Kiwi Shake

THURSDAY
- **Breakfast:** Whole wheat English muffin toasted with Cinnamon Walnut Raisin Low-Fat Cream Cheese; one 8-ounce glass low-fat milk
- **Lunch:** Chicken Tortilla Soup with Spinach
- **Dinner:** Seared Tuna over Confetti Glass Noodle Salad
- **Beauty Snack 1:** Honey Yogurt Cup
- **Beauty Snack 2:** Lemon Sorbet with Fresh Blueberry Sauce

FRIDAY
- **Breakfast:** Spicy Scrambled Breakfast Taco with Tomato Salsa
- **Lunch:** Chicken, Artichoke, Cherry Tomato, and Mozzarella Pasta Toss
- **Dinner:** Oysters Primavera; 2 cups mesclun dressed with 1 teaspoon extra virgin olive oil and 1 tablespoon fresh lemon juice
- **Beauty Snack 1:** Nutty Banana Shake
- **Beauty Snack 2:** Crunchy Dark Chocolate–Dipped Kiwis

SATURDAY
- **Breakfast:** Black and Blue Yogurt Parfait
- **Lunch:** Fire-Roasted Tomato Soup; ½ whole wheat pita with 4 ounces canned tuna, lettuce, tomato, and a squeeze of lemon
- **Dinner:** Grilled Turkey Cutlets with Sweet and Spicy Blueberry Cranberry Relish with Buttermilk Scallion Smashed Sweet Potatoes
- **Beauty Snack 1:** 1 ounce Spiced Walnuts; 1 ounce Parmesan cheese
- **Beauty Snack 2:** Dark Chocolate–Covered Strawberries

SUNDAY

- **Breakfast:** Spinach Omelet; Banana Yogurt Cup
- **Lunch:** Fresh and Fruity Shrimp Salad with Yogurt Dressing; 1 multigrain roll
- **Dinner:** Spiced Salmon with Edamame Succotash
- **Beauty Snack 1:** White Bean "Hummus" with 1 cup each carrot and celery sticks; one 8-ounce glass low-fat milk
- **Beauty Snack 2:** 1 ounce dark chocolate (60 percent cacao) with ½ cup mixed berries; one 8-ounce glass low-fat milk

DAILY AVERAGE FOR WEEK 3

1,500 calories; 106 g protein; 171 g carbohydrates; 23 g fiber; 48 g fat; 14 g saturated fat; 0 trans fats; 290 mg cholesterol; 2,061 mg sodium; 1,035 mg calcium; 3 g omega-3 fats

The Beauty Diet Week 4 Menu (Days 22–28)

MONDAY

- **Breakfast:** Strawberry Raspberry Yogurt Parfait
- **Lunch:** Ginger Teriyaki Salmon Burger
- **Dinner:** Rosemary-Roasted Chicken and Leeks with Slow-Roasted Tomatoes
- **Beauty Snack 1:** 1 ounce Spiced Walnuts; one 8-ounce glass low-fat milk
- **Beauty Snack 2:** Low-Fat Double-Chocolate Milk Shake

TUESDAY

- **Breakfast:** Whole grain English muffin with 2 tablespoons peanut butter; ½ cup blueberries; one 8-ounce glass low-fat milk
- **Lunch:** Baked Crab Cake Pita Sandwich with Spicy Yogurt Sauce

- **Dinner:** Sweet and Crunchy Shrimp–Spinach Salad; one multigrain roll
- **Beauty Snack 1:** Cherry Walnut Granola with Yogurt
- **Beauty Snack 2:** Kiwi and Melon Fruit Soup

WEDNESDAY
- **Breakfast:** Steel-Cut Oats Cooked with Milk, Berries, and Walnuts
- **Lunch:** Salmon Caesar Salad with Tomatoes and Creamy Yogurt Dressing
- **Dinner:** Broiled Oysters Florentine with Mixed Greens
- **Beauty Snack 1:** Quartered Figs Drizzled with Honey Yogurt Sauce and Toasted Almonds; one 8-ounce glass low-fat milk
- **Beauty Snack 2:** 1 ounce dark chocolate (60 percent cacao); 1 cup mixed berries

THURSDAY
- **Breakfast:** Easy Breakfast Sandwich with ½ cup blueberries and strawberries
- **Lunch:** Sweet Potato Bisque with Shrimp and spinach salad
- **Dinner:** Pineapple- and Rum-Marinated Grilled Chicken over Grilled Sweet Potato Salad with Garlicky Wilted Spinach
- **Beauty Snack 1:** Triple-Berry Smoothie; 1 ounce Spiced Walnuts
- **Beauty Snack 2:** Dark Chocolate–Dipped Frozen Bananas

FRIDAY
- **Breakfast:** 1 cup whole grain cereal, such as Kashi GoLean, with ½ cup blueberries and ½ cup low-fat milk
- **Lunch:** Spring Pea and Spinach Soup with Crab; 1 multigrain roll
- **Dinner:** Grilled Striped Bass with Lemony Spinach and Sugar Snap Pea Sauté
- **Beauty Snack 1:** Mango Kiwi Blackberry Smoothie
- **Beauty Snack 2:** Dark Chocolate Brownie with one 8-ounce glass low-fat milk

SATURDAY

- **Breakfast:** Whole Grain Waffles with Apple Raisin Compote and Vanilla Yogurt
- **Lunch:** Turkey, Apple, Spinach, and Caramelized Onion Pressed Sandwich
- **Dinner:** Smoky Shrimp Fajitas with Whole Wheat Tortillas
- **Beauty Snack 1:** 1 ounce Spiced Walnuts; 1 ounce Parmesan cheese
- **Beauty Snack 2:** Dark Chocolate–Dipped Apples with Pistachios

SUNDAY

- **Breakfast:** Sweet Potato, Zucchini, and Goat Cheese Frittata; one 8-ounce glass low-fat milk
- **Lunch:** Grilled Chicken Salad with Blueberries over Spinach in a Honey Balsamic Dressing
- **Dinner:** White Wine–Poached Salmon with Balsamic Roasted Asparagus
- **Beauty Snack 1:** Banana Blueberry Yogurt Cup
- **Beauty Snack 2:** Chocolate Orange Hot Chocolate

DAILY AVERAGE FOR WEEK 4

1,457 calories; 101 g protein; 156 g carbohydrates; 23 g fiber; 52 g fat; 14 g saturated fat; 0 trans fats; 283 mg cholesterol; 1,796 mg sodium; 1,019 mg calcium; 3.7 g omega-3 fats

The Beauty Diet Breakfasts

BANANA BLUEBERRY YOGURT CUP

1 cup low-fat plain yogurt
1 small banana, sliced
½ cup fresh blueberries

Layer the yogurt with the banana slices and blueberries in small bowl.

Yield: 1 serving

Per serving: 286 calories; 15 g protein; 51 g carbohydrates; 4.4 g fiber; 36 g sugars; 4.4 g fat; 2.5 g saturated fat; 0 trans fat; 15 mg cholesterol; 173 mg sodium; 458 mg calcium; 0.1 g omega-3 fats; 230 IU vitamin A; 18 mg vitamin C; 0.6 mg vitamin E; 1 mg iron; 2.5 mg zinc

BANANA YOGURT CUP

1 cup low-fat plain yogurt
¼ cup sliced banana
1 tablespoon wheat germ

Layer the yogurt with the banana slices in a small bowl. Sprinkle with wheat germ.

Yield: 1 serving

Per serving: 215 calories; 15 g protein; 29 g carbohydrates; 2 g fiber; 22 g sugars; 4.7 g fat; 2.6 g saturated fat; 0 trans fat; 15 mg cholesterol; 172 mg sodium; 453 mg calcium; 0.1 g omega-3 fats; 156 IU vitamin A; 6 mg vitamin C; 1.2 mg vitamin E; 1 mg iron; 3.4 mg zinc

CINNAMON WALNUT RAISIN LOW-FAT CREAM CHEESE

4 ounces low-fat cream cheese
½ teaspoon ground cinnamon
8 teaspoons finely chopped toasted walnuts
¼ cup raisins

Blend the cream cheese with the cinnamon, walnuts, and raisins. Refrigerate.

Yield: 4 servings (2 tablespoons cream cheese each)

Per serving: 124 calories; 4 g protein; 11 g carbohydrates; 1 g fiber; 6 g sugars; 8 g fat; 3 g saturated fat; 0 trans fat; 16 mg cholesterol; 85 mg sodium; 45 mg calcium; 0.5 g omega-3 fats; 194 IU vitamin A; 0.4 mg vitamin C; 0.1 mg vitamin E; 1 mg iron; 0.4 mg zinc

EASY BREAKFAST SANDWICH

Nonstick cooking spray
12 egg whites
¼ teaspoon freshly ground black pepper
4 ounces extra-sharp low-fat cheddar cheese, grated
8 slices whole grain bread, toasted
4 slices Canadian bacon, heated
8 thin slices tomato

Heat a medium nonstick skillet sprayed with nonstick cooking spray over medium heat. Add the egg whites, season with pepper, and cook until the whites have firmed, about 3 minutes. Add cheese to firmed whites and cook until cheese has melted. Divide the cheesy egg whites between 4 bread slices and top each with a slice of Canadian bacon, 2 slices of tomato, and a second slice of bread. Cut each sandwich in half and serve.

Yield: 4 servings (1 sandwich each)

Per serving: 305 calories; 32 g protein; 28 g carbohydrates; 5 g fiber; 4.5 g sugars; 6 g fat; 2.4 g saturated fat; 0 trans fat; 19 mg cholesterol; 992 mg sodium; 196 mg calcium; 0.1 g omega-3 fats; 311 IU vitamin A; 4 mg vitamin C; 0.6 mg vitamin E; 2 mg iron; 2 mg zinc

EGG WHITE, SPINACH, AND FETA SCRAMBLE ON WHOLE WHEAT TOAST

8 egg whites (about 1⅓ cups)
¼ teaspoon kosher salt
¼ teaspoon freshly ground black pepper
2 teaspoons water
Nonstick cooking spray
1 cup baby spinach
¼ cup crumbled feta cheese
4 slices whole wheat bread, toasted

Whip the egg whites, salt, pepper, and water in a small bowl until frothy. Spray a nonstick skillet with cooking spray and place over medium heat. Add the egg white mixture and cook, stirring, until almost set. Add the spinach and feta and continue to cook until the eggs are completely cooked and the spinach has wilted. Serve open face on toast.

Yield: 4 servings (about ½ cup egg and 1 slice toast each)

Per serving: 140 calories; 13 g protein; 14 g carbohydrates; 3 g fiber; 2 g sugars; 3 g fat; 1.6 g saturated fat; 0 trans fat; 8 mg cholesterol; 491 mg sodium; 88 mg calcium; 0.03 g omega-3 fats; 255 IU vitamin A; 1 mg vitamin C; 0.2 mg vitamin E; 1 mg iron; 1 mg zinc

FRENCH TOAST STUFFED WITH RICOTTA, KIWI, AND PEACH

1 egg
1 egg white
½ cup low-fat milk
1 teaspoon vanilla extract
3 tablespoons sugar
⅛ teaspoon kosher salt
½ cup part-skim ricotta cheese
¼ cup finely chopped, peeled kiwi
¼ cup finely chopped peach
8 slices whole wheat bread
Nonstick cooking spray

In a medium shallow bowl, whisk together the egg, egg white, milk, vanilla, 2 tablespoons of the sugar, and the salt; set aside. In a small bowl, mix the remaining 1 tablespoon sugar, the ricotta, kiwi, and peach. Divide the ricotta mixture between 4 slices of bread. Top with a second piece of bread and press together firmly. Heat a large nonstick skillet sprayed with nonstick cooking spray. Dip each piece of stuffed French toast into the egg mixture, coating both sides well and letting the excess drip off, and place in the skillet. Cook over medium heat for 2–3 minutes on each side, until well browned and crisped. Serve warm.

Yield: 4 servings (1 piece each)

Per serving: 283 calories; 15 g protein; 41 g carbohydrates; 5 g fiber; 16 g sugars; 6.4 g fat; 2.6 g saturated fat; 0 trans fat; 64 mg cholesterol; 436 mg sodium; 197 mg calcium; 0.05 g omega-3 fats; 286 IU vitamin A; 11 mg vitamin C; 0.7 mg vitamin E; 2 mg iron; 2 mg zinc

OATMEAL WITH CINNAMON, DRIED FRUIT, AND TOASTED WALNUTS

1 cup low-fat milk
2 cups water
¼ teaspoon kosher salt
1 3-inch cinnamon stick
1 cup steel-cut oats
½ cup mixed dried fruit, such as cherries, cranberries, and blueberries
½ cup toasted walnuts, coarsely chopped

In a medium saucepan, bring the milk, water, salt, and cinnamon stick to a boil. Stir in the oats and dried fruit, reduce the heat to low, cover, and cook until tender, about 20 minutes, stirring occasionally to prevent boiling over. Remove the cinnamon stick before serving and top each bowl with 2 tablespoons toasted chopped walnuts.

Yield: 4 servings (scant cup cooked oats each)

Per serving: 322 calories; 11 g protein; 42 g carbohydrates; 6.3 g fiber; 13 g sugars; 13 g fat; 1.8 g saturated fat; 0 trans fat; 3 mg cholesterol; 148 mg sodium; 116 mg calcium; 1.4 g omega-3 fats; 501 IU vitamin A; 0.2 mg vitamin C; 0.4 mg vitamin E; 2.4 mg iron; 2.3 mg zinc

POACHED EGGS FLORENTINE

Nonstick cooking spray
4 cups baby spinach
¼ cup low-fat milk
½ teaspoon cornstarch
¼ cup grated sharp cheddar cheese
2 tablespoons distilled white vinegar
4 eggs
2 whole grain English muffins, split and toasted
¼ teaspoon kosher salt
¼ teaspoon freshly ground black pepper

Spray a small saucepan set over medium high-heat with nonstick cooking spray and add the spinach. Cook until wilted, 2–3 minutes, remove from the pot, and set aside. Add the milk and cornstarch and whisk until smooth. Bring to a simmer, whisking, turn off the heat, add the cheese, and whisk until smooth and thick. Set aside. Bring a medium pot of water to a boil, add the vinegar, and reduce the heat to a bare simmer. Crack the eggs and add one at a time. Let cook until the yolk is set but still soft, 5 minutes. Remove and drain the water. Top each English muffin half with some of the spinach, one poached egg, and some of the cheddar sauce. Season with salt and pepper.

Yield: 4 servings (½ English muffin, ¼ cup cooked spinach, 1 egg, and 2 tablespoons cheese sauce each)

Per serving: 180 calories; 12 g protein; 16 g carbohydrates; 3 g fiber; 4 g sugars; 8 g fat; 3 g saturated fat; 0 trans fat; 219 mg cholesterol; 493 mg sodium; 209 mg calcium; 0.1 g omega-3 fats; 2,689 IU vitamin A; 7 mg vitamin C; 1.2 mg vitamin E; 2.5 mg iron; 1.5 mg zinc

SCRAMBLED EGG WHITES WITH CHEDDAR AND TOMATO AND SLICED KIWI

8 large egg whites
¼ teaspoon kosher salt
¼ teaspoon freshly ground black pepper
2 teaspoons water
Nonstick cooking spray
¼ cup grated sharp white cheddar cheese

⅓ cup diced tomato
2 tablespoons chopped fresh chives
4 kiwis, peeled and sliced

Whip the egg whites, salt, pepper, and water in a small bowl until frothy. Spray a nonstick skillet with cooking spray and place over medium heat. Add the egg white mixture and cook, stirring, until almost set. Add the cheese, tomato, and chives and continue to cook until the eggs are set and the cheese is melted. Divide the scrambled eggs and sliced kiwi evenly among four plates.

Yield: 4 servings (⅓ cup egg scramble and 1 kiwi each)

Per serving: 114 calories; 10 g protein; 13 g carbohydrates; 2.5 g fiber; 7.8 g sugars; 2.8 g fat; 1.3 g saturated fat; 0 g trans fat; 7.5 mg cholesterol; 327 mg sodium; 83 mg calcium; 0.03 g omega-3 fats; 290 IU vitamin A; 74 mg vitamin C; 1.1 mg vitamin E; 0.4 mg iron; 0.1 mg zinc

SPICY SCRAMBLED BREAKFAST TACO WITH TOMATO SALSA

Nonstick cooking spray
4 eggs
4 egg whites
¼ teaspoon kosher salt
¼ teaspoon freshly ground black pepper
¼ teaspoon chili powder
2 scallions, sliced
1½ ounces grated sharp cheddar cheese
4 8-inch flour tortillas, warmed
½ cup tomato salsa

Heat a medium nonstick skillet sprayed with nonstick cooking spray over medium-high heat. Beat the eggs, egg whites, salt, pepper, and chili powder in a medium bowl. Add to the skillet and cook, stirring, until just set. Add the scallions and cheese and cook for another minute or until the cheese is melted. Divide the eggs evenly among the tortillas, top with salsa, and roll.

Yield: 4 servings (1 taco each)

Per serving: 300 calories; 17 g protein; 28 g carbohydrates; 2.2 g fiber; 1.8 g sugars; 12 g fat; 4.7 g saturated fat; 0 trans fat; 222 mg cholesterol; 748 mg sodium; 178 mg calcium; 0.1 g omega-3 fats; 629 IU vitamin A; 3 mg vitamin C; 1 mg vitamin E; 3.4 mg iron; 1.2 mg zinc

SPINACH OMELET

16 egg whites
2 tablespoons water
¼ teaspoon kosher salt
¼ teaspoon freshly ground black pepper
Nonstick cooking spray
1 cup finely chopped onion
2 cups baby spinach, roughly chopped

In a medium bowl, whisk together the egg whites, water, salt, and pepper; set aside. Heat a large nonstick skillet sprayed with cooking spray over medium heat. Add the onion and cook until softened, 3–5 minutes. Add the spinach and cook until wilted, 1 minute. Add the egg mixture and cook until the edges are set and the top is no longer runny, about 4–5 minutes. Fold in half and cook for an additional 2 minutes on each side. Cut into 4 wedges and serve.

Yield: 4 servings (¼ omelet each)

Per serving: 91 calories; 15 g protein; 5 g carbohydrates; 1 g fiber; 3 g sugars; 0.5 g fat; 0 saturated fat; 0 trans fat; 0 cholesterol; 354 mg sodium; 32 mg calcium; 0.02 g omega-3 fats; 1,173 IU vitamin A; 6.5 mg vitamin C; 0.3 mg vitamin E; 0.6 mg iron; 0.2 mg zinc

STEEL-CUT OATS COOKED WITH MILK, BERRIES, AND WALNUTS

½ cup skim milk
2½ cups water
¼ teaspoon salt
1 cup steel-cut oats
1 cup mixed berries, such as blueberries, raspberries, and sliced
    strawberries
¼ cup toasted chopped walnuts

In a medium saucepan, bring the milk, water, and salt to a boil. Stir in the oats, reduce the heat to low, cover, and cook, stirring occasionally, until tender, about 20 minutes. Top each bowl with ¼ cup mixed berries and 1 tablespoon chopped walnuts.

Yield: 4 servings (about ¾ cup cooked oats each)

Per serving: 214 calories; 8.5 g protein; 34 g carbohydrates; 6 g fiber; 3.6 g sugars; 7.4 g fat; 1 g saturated fat; 0 trans fat; 0 cholesterol; 162 mg sodium; 63 mg calcium; 0.7 g omega-3 fats; 72 IU vitamin A; 11.5 mg vitamin C; 0.2 mg vitamin E; 2 mg iron; 0.3 mg zinc

STRAWBERRY RASPBERRY YOGURT PARFAIT

1 cup sliced strawberries
1 cup raspberries
1 tablespoon sugar
1½ teaspoons vanilla extract
2⅔ cups low-fat plain yogurt
8 teaspoons wheat germ

Combine the strawberries, raspberries, and sugar in a medium bowl. Let sit at room temperature for 5–10 minutes or until the berries become juicy. Meanwhile, stir the vanilla extract into the yogurt. To assemble each parfait, layer ⅓ cup yogurt, 1 teaspoon wheat germ, ¼ cup berries, and repeat.

Yield: 4 parfaits (1 parfait each)

Per serving: 159 calories; 10.5 g protein; 24 g carbohydrates; 3.5 g fiber; 16 g sugars; 3 g fat; 1.7 g saturated fat; 0 trans fat; 10 mg cholesterol; 115 mg sodium; 313 mg calcium; 0.1 g omega-3 fats; 93 IU vitamin A; 32 mg vitamin C; 1 mg vitamin E; 1 mg iron; 2.3 mg zinc

SWEET POTATO, ZUCCHINI, AND GOAT CHEESE FRITTATA

1 tablespoon extra virgin olive oil
1 medium sweet potato, peeled and thinly sliced
1 small zucchini, thinly sliced
½ teaspoon kosher salt
¼ teaspoon freshly ground black pepper
4 eggs
4 egg whites
1 teaspoon chopped fresh thyme
2 tablespoons water
2 ounces fresh goat cheese, broken into small pieces

Preheat the oven to 450°F. Heat the oil in a medium nonstick skillet set over medium heat. Add potato and zucchini slices, spread into an even layer, and cook, undisturbed, for 5 minutes or until the potatoes turn bright orange and begin to soften. Stir, season with ¼ teaspoon of the salt and the pepper, and continue to cook until the potatoes are tender and lightly browned. Meanwhile, in a medium bowl, whip the eggs, egg whites, remaining ¼ teaspoon salt, thyme, and water until well mixed and frothy. Pour over the vegetables and cook until the edges are set, 5 minutes. Sprinkle the goat cheese evenly over the frittata, place in the oven, and cook until the eggs are set and puffed. Let cool for 5 minutes and slice.

Yield: 4 servings (¼ frittata each)

Per serving: 190 calories; 13 g protein; 8 g carbohydrates; 1.3 g fiber; 3 g sugars; 11 g fat; 4 g saturated fat; 0 trans fat; 218 mg cholesterol; 429 mg sodium; 64 mg calcium; 0.1 g omega-3 fats; 6,414 IU vitamin A; 7 mg vitamin C; 1.3 mg vitamin E; 1.7 mg iron; 1 mg zinc

TOMATO SCALLION FRITTATA WITH TURKEY BACON

Nonstick cooking spray
1 medium tomato, diced
3 scallions, green part only, cut into 1-inch pieces
4 eggs
4 egg whites
¼ cup low-fat milk

¼ teaspoon kosher salt
¼ teaspoon freshly ground black pepper
8 slices turkey bacon, cooked

Preheat the oven to 425°F. Heat a medium ovenproof nonstick skillet sprayed with nonstick cooking spray over medium heat. Add the tomato and scallions and sauté until warmed through and some of the tomato liquid has evaporated, 5 minutes. Meanwhile, beat the eggs, egg whites, milk, salt, and pepper until well mixed and slightly frothy. Pour over the tomato and scallions and cook until the edges are just set, about 3 minutes. Transfer to the oven and cook until puffed and browned and the eggs are set, 12–15 minutes. Let cool slightly, turn out of the skillet, and cut into 4 wedges. Serve each wedge with 2 slices of turkey bacon.

Yield: 4 servings (¼ frittata and 2 slices bacon each)

Per serving: 216 calories; 19 g protein; 5 g carbohydrates; 1 g fiber; 2.6 g sugars; 13 g fat; 4 g saturated fat; 0 trans fat; 240 mg cholesterol; 904 mg sodium; 62 mg calcium; 0.2 g omega-3 fats; 696 IU vitamin A; 7 mg vitamin C; 1 mg vitamin E; 2 mg iron; 2 mg zinc

TRIPLE-BERRY SMOOTHIE

2 cups halved strawberries
½ cup raspberries
½ cup blueberries
2 tablespoons honey
½ teaspoon grated fresh lemon zest
1 cup low-fat plain yogurt

Combine all the ingredients in a blender and blend until smooth. Serve over ice if desired.

Yield: 4 servings (approximately 1 cup each)

Per serving: 116 calories; 4 g protein; 24 g carbohydrates; 3 g fiber; 18 g sugars; 1 g fat; 0.6 g saturated fat; 0 trans fat; 3.7 mg cholesterol; 44 mg sodium; 129 mg calcium; 0.1 g omega-3 fats; 51 IU vitamin A; 54 mg vitamin C; 0.4 mg vitamin E; 0.5 mg iron; 0.7 mg zinc

WHOLE GRAIN BLUEBERRY PANCAKES

1 cup buckwheat pancake mix, such as Bob's Red Mill
½ cup buttermilk
1 egg
⅓ cup water
½ teaspoon grated lemon zest
⅛ teaspoon kosher salt
Nonstick cooking spray
1 cup blueberries
½ cup pure maple syrup

In a medium bowl, combine the pancake mix, buttermilk, egg, water, lemon zest, and salt. Whisk until just combined. Heat a medium non-stick skillet sprayed with nonstick cooking spray over medium-high heat and drop ¼ cup of batter at a time into the skillet. When the edges of the pancakes are set, after 3 minutes, sprinkle about 2 tablespoons blueberries into the wet side of each pancake and flip. Continue to cook until just cooked through, 2 minutes. Repeat with the remaining batter. Serve with maple syrup.

Yield: 4 servings (2 large pancakes each)

Per serving: 260 calories; 7 g protein; 52 g carbohydrates; 3 g fiber; 31 g sugars; 3 g fat; 0.8 g saturated fat; 0 trans fat; 56 mg cholesterol; 469 mg sodium; 147 mg calcium; 0.03 g omega-3 fats; 89 IU vitamin A; 4 mg vitamin C; 0.4 mg vitamin E; 2 mg iron; 2 mg zinc

WHOLE GRAIN WAFFLES WITH APPLE RAISIN COMPOTE AND VANILLA YOGURT

8 frozen whole grain waffles, such as Kashi GoLean Waffles
¼ cup raisins
2 tablespoons water
1 tablespoon butter
2 small apples, peeled, cored, and sliced
2 tablespoons light brown sugar
1 cup low-fat plain yogurt
¼ teaspoon vanilla extract

Heat the waffles according to the package directions and keep warm. In a small microwave-safe dish, mix the raisins and water and microwave for 1 minute, until the raisins plump. Heat the butter in a small skillet over medium heat and add the apples and brown sugar. Cook until the apples are tender, 5 minutes, and then add the raisins. Remove from the heat. Combine the yogurt and vanilla and top the waffles with the apple compote and vanilla yogurt.

Yield: 4 servings (2 waffles, about ½ cup apple compote, and ¼ cup yogurt each)

Per serving: 314 calories; 12 g protein; 58 g carbohydrates; 7 g fiber; 26 g sugars; 7 g fat; 2.4 g saturated fat; 0 trans fat; 11 mg cholesterol; 396 mg sodium; 186 mg calcium; 0.02 g omega-3 fats; 137 IU vitamin A; 3 mg vitamin C; 0.1 mg vitamin E; 2 mg iron; 1 mg zinc

The Beauty Diet Lunches

ANYTIME THANKSGIVING SALAD

Sage Vinaigrette
¼ cup white wine vinegar
¼ teaspoon kosher salt
¼ teaspoon freshly ground black pepper
1 tablespoon chopped fresh sage
2 tablespoons extra virgin olive oil

Salad
12 ounces roasted turkey breast, diced
¼ cup dried cranberries
¼ cup toasted chopped pecans
8 cups baby spinach

Make the vinaigrette by whisking together all the ingredients except the oil until well combined. Slowly whisk in the oil until incorporated. Set aside.

In a large bowl, combine all the salad ingredients. Pour the dressing over the salad and toss well to coat.

Yield: 4 servings (about 2 cups each)

Per serving: 268 calories; 27 g protein; 12 g carbohydrates; 3.4 g fiber; 5 g sugars; 12.6 g fat; 1.6 g saturated fat; 0 trans fat; 70 mg cholesterol; 242 mg sodium; 53 mg calcium; 0.13 g omega-3 fats; 1,729 IU vitamin A; 7 mg vitamin C; 1.1 mg vitamin E; 3.1 mg iron; 2 mg zinc

ARTICHOKE BRUSCHETTA SALAD

3 slices whole wheat bread
1 large clove garlic, cut in half
1 6-ounce jar marinated artichoke hearts, drained
2 medium tomatoes, diced
1 10.5-ounce can white beans, drained and rinsed
1 small red onion, thinly sliced
8 ounces roasted turkey breast, diced
8 cups mesclun
¼ cup fresh lemon juice
¼ teaspoon kosher salt
¼ teaspoon freshly ground black pepper
2 tablespoons extra virgin olive oil

Preheat the oven to 400°F. Place the bread on a baking sheet and toast in the oven until lightly browned and crisped, 10 minutes. Immediately rub with the garlic clove while hot and then set aside to cool and crisp further.

In a large bowl, mix the artichoke hearts, diced tomatoes, white beans, red onion, diced turkey, and greens. Add the lemon juice, salt, and pepper and toss to combine well. Cut the garlic croutons into 1- to 2-inch cubes and add to the bowl. Drizzle the olive oil into the bowl and give everything one final toss.

Yield: 4 servings (2 generous cups each)

Per serving: 338 calories; 28 g protein; 36 g carbohydrates; 9 g fiber; 5 g sugars; 10.5 g fat; 1.4 g saturated fat; 0 trans fat; 47 mg cholesterol; 713 mg sodium; 150 mg calcium; 0.1 g omega-3 fats; 1,645 IU vitamin A; 28 mg vitamin C; 2 mg vitamin E; 5 mg iron; 3 mg zinc

BAKED CRAB CAKE PITA SANDWICHES WITH SPICY YOGURT SAUCE

Crab Cakes
½ pound lump crabmeat, picked over for shells
1 egg
1 tablespoon Dijon mustard
½ teaspoon hot sauce, such as Frank's RedHot sauce
2 teaspoons fresh lemon juice
2 tablespoons chopped fresh parsley leaves
2 tablespoons chopped scallion
½ cup panko, plus ⅓ cup for dredging
¼ teaspoon kosher salt
½ teaspoon freshly ground black pepper

Spicy Yogurt Sauce
¼ cup low-fat plain yogurt
1 teaspoon fresh lemon juice
½ teaspoon hot sauce, such as Frank's RedHot sauce
1 tablespoon chopped fresh parsley

Sandwiches
4 romaine leaves, chopped coarse
2 medium tomatoes, sliced ¼ inch thick
4 whole wheat pita pockets

Preheat the oven to 450° and line a baking sheet with aluminum foil. In a medium bowl, combine the crab, egg, mustard, hot sauce, lemon juice, parsley, scallion, ½ cup panko, ¼ teaspoon salt, and ½ teaspoon freshly ground black pepper. Form into 4 equal patties and coat in the ⅓ cup panko on both sides. Place on the prepared baking sheet and bake for 15–20 minutes or until heated through and lightly browned. Let cool slightly.

Meanwhile, in a small bowl, combine all the ingredients for the spicy yogurt sauce. To assemble, divide chopped lettuce and sliced tomato equally among the pita pockets. Top with 1 crab cake and a heaping tablespoon yogurt sauce.

Yield: 4 servings (1 sandwich each)

Per serving: 324 calories; 23 g protein; 50 g carbohydrates; 7 g fiber; 4 g sugars; 5 g fat; 1 g saturated fat; 0 trans fat; 110 mg cholesterol; 836 mg sodium; 126 mg calcium; 0.3 g omega-3 fats; 1,568 IU vitamin A; 20 mg vitamin C; 2 mg vitamin E; 3.5 mg iron; 4 mg zinc

CALIFORNIA TURKEY BURGER WITH CREAMY AVOCADO YOGURT SPREAD

1 pound ground turkey
½ teaspoon kosher salt
¼ teaspoon freshly ground black pepper
¼ teaspoon chili powder
2 tablespoons barbecue sauce
1 ripe avocado
2 tablespoons low-fat plain yogurt
4 whole wheat hamburger buns
4 romaine lettuce leaves
¼ cup thinly sliced red onion

Preheat the broiler and line a baking sheet with aluminum foil. Gently mix the ground turkey, ¼ teaspoon of the salt, the pepper, and the chili powder in a medium bowl until well combined and divide into four equal patties. Place on the prepared baking sheet and brush with barbecue sauce. Place under the broiler and cook for 5–7 minutes on each side or until just cooked through. Meanwhile, peel, pit, and mash the avocado with the yogurt and the remaining ¼ teaspoon salt. Assemble the burgers by lightly toasting the buns and place the lettuce and onion on the bottom bun, top with 1 burger patty, avocado spread, and the top bun.

Yield: 4 servings (1 burger each)

Per serving: 398 calories; 27 g protein; 30 g carbohydrates; 7 g fiber; 7 g sugars; 19 g fat; 4 g saturated fat; 0 trans fat; 82 mg cholesterol; 632 mg sodium; 93 mg calcium; 0.3 g omega-3 fats; 715 IU vitamin A; 7 mg vitamin C; 2 mg vitamin E; 3 mg iron; 3.6 mg zinc

CHICKEN, ARTICHOKE, CHERRY TOMATO, AND MOZZARELLA PASTA TOSS

8 ounces dried penne pasta
Nonstick cooking spray
1 pound boneless, skinless chicken breasts
½ teaspoon kosher salt
¼ teaspoon freshly ground black pepper
¼ teaspoon hot red pepper flakes
1 cup grape tomatoes, halved
1 6-ounce jar marinated artichoke hearts, drained well
4 ounces fresh mozzarella cheese, cubed
1 tablespoon white wine vinegar
2 tablespoons chopped fresh chives

Preheat the broiler. Bring a large pot of water to a boil and cook the pasta according to the package directions; drain well and keep warm. Meanwhile, spray a foil-lined baking sheet with nonstick cooking spray and lay the chicken on top. Season with ¼ teaspoon of the salt, the pepper, and the hot red pepper flakes. Broil until just cooked through, 8–10 minutes. Let cool slightly, dice, and combine in a large bowl with the cooked pasta, tomatoes, artichoke hearts, mozzarella, remaining ¼ teaspoon salt, vinegar, and chives.

Yield: 4 servings (about 2 cups each)

Per serving: 441 calories; 36.5 g protein; 48 g carbohydrates; 4 g fiber; 3 g sugars; 12 g fat; 4.6 g saturated fat; 0 trans fat; 85 mg cholesterol; 402 mg sodium; 143 mg calcium; 0.1 g omega-3 fats; 640 IU vitamin A; 9 mg vitamin C; 0.5 mg vitamin E; 3.2 mg iron; 2 mg zinc

CHICKEN TORTILLA SOUP WITH SPINACH

1 tablespoon extra virgin olive oil
1 cup chopped onion
1 jalapeño chile, seeded and minced
1 teaspoon cumin seeds
1 14.5-ounce can low-sodium chicken broth
1 cup water
1 pound boneless, skinless chicken breast
1 14.5-ounce can white hominy, drained
2 cups baby spinach
1 to 2 tablespoons fresh lime juice, to taste
2 tablespoons chopped fresh cilantro
2 cups crushed baked tortilla chips for garnish

Heat the olive oil in a large saucepan over medium-high heat. Add the onion, jalapeño, and cumin and sauté until the onion is tender, 3–5 minutes. Add the chicken broth and water and bring to a simmer. Add the chicken and simmer until just cooked through, 10 minutes. Remove the chicken and cool slightly; shred. Meanwhile, add the hominy and baby spinach and cook until the hominy is warmed through and the spinach is wilted. Add the shredded chicken back to the pot and season with lime juice and cilantro. Garnish each bowl with ½ cup of the tortilla chips.

Yield: 4 servings (1¼ cups soup and ½ cup tortilla chips each)

Per serving: 387 calories; 33 g protein; 38 g carbohydrates; 4.5 g fiber; 3 g sugars; 11 g fat; 2 g saturated fat; 0 trans fat; 66 mg cholesterol; 563 mg sodium; 101 mg calcium; 0.1 g omega-3 fats; 1,295 IU vitamin A; 12 mg vitamin C; 2 mg vitamin E; 3 mg iron; 2.2 mg zinc

CURRY CHICKEN SALAD OVER BABY SPINACH

1½ pounds thinly sliced boneless, skinless chicken breast
½ cup plus 2 tablespoons nonfat plain yogurt
1¼ teaspoons curry powder
1 teaspoon salt
¼ teaspoon cayenne
¼ cup white wine vinegar
⅔ cup finely diced apple
⅔ cup finely diced celery
½ cup finely diced sweet onion
8 cups baby spinach

Place the oven rack about 6 inches from the broiler and preheat the broiler. Line a baking sheet with aluminum foil and set aside. In a small bowl, combine the chicken, 2 tablespoons of the yogurt, ½ teaspoon of the curry powder, ½ teaspoon of the salt, the cayenne, and 2 tablespoons of the white wine vinegar. Marinate at room temperature for 10 minutes. Lay on the prepared baking sheet in a single layer and place under the broiler for about 4 minutes per side or until just cooked through. Let cool slightly and then dice. Combine the cooked chicken with the apple, celery, and onion. In a small bowl, stir together the remaining ½ cup yogurt, ¾ teaspoon curry powder, ½ teaspoon salt, and 2 tablespoons white wine vinegar. Pour the dressing over the chicken mixture, toss well, and serve over baby spinach.

Yield: 4 servings (1 cup chicken salad and 2 cups spinach each)

Per serving: 230 calories; 38 g protein; 10 g carbohydrates; 2 g fiber; 5 g sugars; 4 g fat; 1 g saturated fat; 0 trans fat; 95 mg cholesterol; 740 mg sodium; 127 mg calcium; 0.1 g omega-3 fats; 4,880 IU vitamin A; 18 mg vitamin C; 2 mg vitamin E; 3 mg iron; 1.5 mg zinc

FIRE-ROASTED TOMATO SOUP

1½ pounds plum tomatoes
1 small onion, peeled and cut into 6 wedges
2 cloves garlic
1 tablespoon extra virgin olive oil
¼ teaspoon kosher salt
¼ teaspoon freshly ground black pepper
2 teaspoons thyme leaves
1 14.5-ounce can vegetable broth

Preheat the broiler. Core and halve the tomatoes and place in a bowl with the onion and garlic. Toss with the oil, salt, and pepper. Place on a baking sheet and broil until softened and charred, 12–15 minutes. Let cool slightly; then place in a blender with the thyme leaves and puree until slightly chunky. Pour into a saucepan, add the broth, and bring to a boil. Simmer until thickened, 25 minutes.

Yield: 4 servings (about 1¼ cups each)

Per serving: 80 calories; 2 g protein; 11 g carbohydrates; 3 g fiber; 6 g sugars; 4 g fat; 0.5 g saturated fat; 0 trans fat; 0 cholesterol; 190 mg sodium; 35 mg calcium; 0.03 g omega-3 fats; 1,309 IU vitamin A; 23 mg vitamin C; 1.3 mg vitamin E; 1 mg iron; 0.3 mg zinc

FRESH AND FRUITY SHRIMP SALAD WITH YOGURT DRESSING

1 lemon
½ teaspoon kosher salt
1 pound peeled and deveined jumbo shrimp (21–25 count)
1 cup diced mango
1 cup sliced strawberries
1 cup sliced seedless cucumber
8 cups mesclun greens
¼ cup low-fat plain yogurt
1 tablespoon apple cider vinegar
1 tablespoon minced shallot
2 teaspoons poppy seeds

Bring a large pot of water to a boil. Halve the lemon, squeeze the juice into the water, and add the whole lemon halves and ¼ teaspoon of the salt. Add the shrimp and simmer until just cooked through, 5 minutes. Drain well, cool, and set aside. In a large bowl, combine the mango, strawberries, cucumber, and greens. Add the shrimp. In a small bowl, stir together the yogurt, vinegar, shallot, poppy seeds, and remaining ¼ teaspoon salt. Pour over the salad and toss well.

Yield: 4 servings (about 2 cups each)

Per serving: 166 calories; 21 g protein; 16 g carbohydrates; 3.3 g fiber; 10 g sugars; 2.2 g fat; 0.6 g saturated fat; 0 trans fat; 169 mg cholesterol; 220 mg sodium; 142 mg calcium; 0.3 g omega-3 fats; 1,599 IU vitamin A; 46 mg vitamin C; 2 mg vitamin E; 4 mg iron; 2 mg zinc

GINGER TERIYAKI SALMON BURGER

1½ pounds skinless wild salmon
1 1-inch piece fresh ginger, grated
2 cloves garlic, grated
2 scallions, chopped
1 tablespoon teriyaki sauce
1 tablespoon hoisin sauce
2 egg whites
1½ tablespoons extra virgin olive oil
4 whole wheat hamburger buns, toasted
4 slices tomato
4 lettuce leaves

Finely chop the salmon until slightly chunky or pulse 3–5 times in a food processor and place in a medium bowl. Add the ginger, garlic, scallions, teriyaki sauce, hoisin sauce, and egg whites. Mix well. Heat the oil in a large skillet over medium-high heat. Form 4 patties and place in the hot oil. Cook, without pressing down, until well browned, 5 minutes. Flip and continue to cook until the patties are just cooked through, 5 minutes. Top each hamburger bun with tomato, lettuce, and 1 salmon patty.

Yield: 4 servings (1 burger each)

Per serving: 469 calories; 45 g protein; 27 g carbohydrates; 4 g fiber; 6 g sugars; 19 g fat; 3 g saturated fat; 0 trans fat; 107 mg cholesterol; 560 mg sodium; 86 mg calcium; 3.5 g omega-3 fats; 1,048 IU vitamin A; 6 mg vitamin C; 3 mg vitamin E; 3 mg iron; 2.2 mg zinc

GREEK TUNA AND SPINACH SALAD WITH YOGURT DILL DRESSING

Yogurt Dill Dressing
¼ cup low-fat plain yogurt
1 tablespoon apple cider vinegar
¼ teaspoon kosher salt
¼ teaspoon freshly ground black pepper
2 tablespoons chopped fresh dill

Salad

1 6-ounce can solid light tuna in olive oil, drained
1 10.5-ounce can chickpeas, drained
¼ cup garlic-stuffed olives, roughly chopped
1 7.5-ounce jar roasted red peppers, drained and sliced
1 cup sliced seedless cucumber
⅓ cup crumbled feta
6 cups baby spinach

Combine all the dressing ingredients in a small bowl and mix well. Set aside. In a large bowl, combine all the salad ingredients and toss well with dressing

Yield: 4 servings (2 cups dressed salad each)

Per serving: 224 calories; 16 g protein; 22 g carbohydrates; 5 g fiber; 3.5 g sugars; 8 g fat; 3 g saturated fat; 0 trans fat; 32 mg cholesterol; 899 mg sodium; 169 mg calcium; 0.2 g omega-3 fats; 3,596 IU vitamin A; 41 mg vitamin C; 1.1 mg vitamin E; 3 mg iron; 2 mg zinc

GRILLED CHICKEN SALAD WITH BLUEBERRIES OVER SPINACH IN A HONEY BALSAMIC DRESSING

Dressing

1 tablespoon honey
1 tablespoon Dijon mustard
¼ teaspoon kosher salt
1 tablespoon balsamic vinegar
1 tablespoon extra virgin olive oil

Salad

1 pound thinly sliced boneless, skinless chicken breasts
¼ teaspoon kosher salt
1 tablespoon fresh lemon juice
8 cups baby spinach
1 cup blueberries
1 cup sliced cucumber
2 tablespoons chopped fresh chives

Preheat a grill for cooking over direct heat or heat a grill pan over medium-high heat. Prepare the dressing by whisking the honey, Dijon mustard, salt, and balsamic vinegar in a small bowl until well combined. Continue to whisk while drizzling in the oil until combined. Set aside. Season the chicken with salt and lemon juice and grill until just cooked through, 3–5 minutes on each side. Let cool slightly and slice. Top the spinach with blueberries, cucumber, sliced chicken, chopped chives, and dressing. Toss well.

Yield: 4 servings (about 2½ cups each)

Per serving: 214 calories; 25 g protein; 14 g carbohydrates; 2 g fiber; 9 g sugars; 6.5 g fat; 1 g saturated fat; 0 trans fat; 62 mg cholesterol; 429 mg sodium; 68 mg calcium; 0.2 g omega-3 fats; 4,629 IU vitamin A; 21 mg vitamin C; 2 mg vitamin E; 2.3 mg iron; 1.1 mg zinc

GRILLED CHICKEN SANDWICH WITH WALNUT BASIL PESTO AND MOZZARELLA

Pesto
1½ cups packed fresh basil leaves
1 small clove garlic
½ teaspoon kosher salt
½ teaspoon freshly ground black pepper
1 tablespoon extra virgin olive oil
2 tablespoons chopped walnuts

Sandwich
Nonstick cooking spray
1 pound thinly sliced boneless, skinless chicken breast
8 slices whole grain bread
4 ounces part-skim mozzarella cheese, sliced

In the bowl of a small food processor, combine the basil, garlic, half of the salt and pepper, and the oil and pulse until chopped and combined. Add the walnuts and pulse 3–5 times, until the nuts are incorporated but the mixture is still chunky. Set aside.

Heat a grill for cooking over direct heat or a grill pan sprayed with nonstick cooking spray over medium-high heat. Season the chicken with the remaining salt and pepper and grill for 4–6 minutes on each side or until just cooked through. Toast the bread and assemble the sandwiches. Top one slice of bread with chicken, pesto, mozzarella, and then a second piece of bread. Repeat to make 4 sandwiches.

Yield: 4 servings (1 sandwich each)

Per serving: 423 calories; 40 g protein; 29 g carbohydrates; 6 g fiber; 3 g sugars; 16 g fat; 5.5 g saturated fat; 0 trans fat; 78 mg cholesterol; 738 mg sodium; 322 mg calcium; 0.5 g omega-3 fats; 1,283 IU vitamin A; 4 mg vitamin C; 1 mg vitamin E; 3.2 mg iron; 3 mg zinc

HAM, ZUCCHINI, RED ONION, SPINACH, AND RICOTTA PANINI

Nonstick cooking spray
1 zucchini, halved crosswise and sliced lengthwise ¼ inch thick
8 slices whole wheat bread
¾ cup part-skim ricotta cheese
1 cup thinly sliced red onion
8 ounces thinly sliced deli honey ham
1½ cups baby spinach

Heat a medium nonstick skillet sprayed with nonstick cooking spray over medium heat. Add the zucchini slices and cook until lightly browned and wilted, about 5 minutes. Transfer to a paper towel–lined plate to cool. Lay out 4 slices of bread and top with equal amounts of ricotta cheese, sliced onion, honey ham, baby spinach, and zucchini slices. Top each sandwich with another slice of bread. Spray the same skillet with nonstick cooking spray, set over medium heat, and cook each sandwich, pressing lightly, until the bread is toasted and golden brown, 3 minutes.

Yield: 4 servings (1 panini each)

Per serving: 312 calories; 25 g protein; 37 g carbohydrates; 6 g fiber; 5 g sugars; 7.6 g fat; 3 g saturated fat; 0 trans fat; 27 mg cholesterol; 870 mg sodium; 219 mg calcium; 0.1 g omega-3 fats; 1,232 IU vitamin A; 9.4 mg vitamin C; 1 mg vitamin E; 2.5 mg iron; 2.4 mg zinc

HUMMUS AND GRILLED VEGETABLE WRAP

1 red bell pepper, quartered
1 yellow bell pepper, quartered
1 large sweet onion, cut into ½-inch-thick rings
1 small zucchini, cut into ¼-inch-thick slices
1 small eggplant, sliced into ½-inch-thick rounds
1 tablespoon extra virgin olive oil
¼ teaspoon kosher salt
½ teaspoon hot red pepper flakes
4 8-inch tortilla wraps
1 recipe White Bean "Hummus" (see Index)
2 cups baby spinach

Heat a large nonstick grill pan over medium-high heat. Toss the bell peppers, onion, zucchini, and eggplant in a large bowl with the olive oil, salt, and hot red pepper flakes. Place on the grill, in batches if necessary, and cook until well marked and softened, 5 to 10 minutes. Transfer the vegetables to a large plate as they are done. Slice the bell pepper quarters into strips and assemble the wraps: spread an equal amount of hummus on each tortilla and top with baby spinach and grilled vegetables. Roll each wrap tightly and cut in half at an angle.

Yield: 4 servings (1 wrap each)

Per serving: 422 calories; 15 g protein; 67 g carbohydrates; 13 g fiber; 14 g sugars; 10 g fat; 0.8 g saturated fat; 0 trans fat; 0 cholesterol; 714 mg sodium; 121 mg calcium; 0.2 g omega-3 fats; 2,384 IU vitamin A; 112 mg vitamin C; 2 mg vitamin E; 4 mg iron; 1.2 mg zinc

LEMON-GRILLED CHICKEN OVER MIXED GREEN SALAD WITH YOGURT DILL DRESSING

Dressing
¼ cup low-fat plain yogurt
1 tablespoon apple cider vinegar
¼ teaspoon kosher salt
¼ teaspoon freshly ground black pepper
2 tablespoons chopped fresh dill

Grilled Chicken
Nonstick cooking spray
12 ounces boneless, skinless chicken tenderloins
1 lemon
¼ teaspoon kosher salt
¼ teaspoon freshly ground black pepper

Salad
4 cups baby spinach
1 cup sliced seedless cucumber
1 6-ounce jar marinated artichoke hearts, drained
1 medium tomato, chopped (½ cup)

To prepare the dressing, stir all the ingredients together in a small bowl. Set aside.

Preheat a grill for cooking over direct heat or a grill pan over medium-high heat and spray with nonstick cooking spray. Place the chicken in a medium bowl and squeeze the lemon all over the chicken. Season with ¼ teaspoon each salt and pepper. Grill until just cooked through, about 4 minutes on each side. Set aside to cool.

In a large bowl, mix the baby spinach, cucumber, artichokes, and tomato and toss well with half of the prepared dressing. Divide among four plates; top with equal amounts of chicken and the remaining dressing and serve.

Yield: 4 servings (1¼ cups dressed salad and 3 ounces chicken each)

Per serving: 143 calories; 19 g protein; 8 g carbohydrates; 2.3 g fiber; 2.9 g sugars; 4.5 g fat; 0.8 g saturated fat; 0 trans fat; 48 mg cholesterol; 396 mg sodium; 72 mg calcium; 0.1 g omega-3 fats; 2,725 IU vitamin A; 18 mg vitamin C; 1 mg vitamin E; 1.5 mg iron; 1 mg zinc

LIME- AND CILANTRO-MARINATED CHICKEN

1½ pounds boneless, skinless chicken breast
2 cloves garlic, smashed
1 teaspoon whole cumin
½ sweet onion, sliced
5 sprigs fresh cilantro
½ lime
¼ teaspoon kosher salt
¼ teaspoon freshly ground black pepper

In a resealable plastic bag, combine the chicken, garlic, cumin, onion, and cilantro. Squeeze the lime directly into the bag and add the squeezed lime. Seal, shake the bag well, and marinate in the refrigerator for 1–2 hours. Preheat the oven to 425°F. Remove the chicken from the marinade and place on an aluminum foil–lined baking sheet. Season with salt and pepper and roast until just cooked through, 12–15 minutes. Let rest for 5 minutes, slice, and serve.

Yield: 4 servings (6 ounces each)

Per serving: 202 calories; 35 g protein; 4.5 g carbohydrates; 0.5 g fiber; 2 g sugars; 4 g fat; 1 g saturated fat; 0 trans fat; 94 mg cholesterol; 207 mg sodium; 34 mg calcium; 0.1 g omega-3 fats; 67 IU vitamin A; 5 mg vitamin C; 0.4 mg vitamin E; 2 mg iron; 1.2 mg zinc

LOBSTER SALAD SANDWICH WITH A CREAMY YOGURT DRESSING

Dressing
⅓ cup low-fat plain yogurt
2 teaspoons fresh lemon juice
¼ teaspoon cayenne pepper, or to taste
1 tablespoon chopped fresh parsley
1 tablespoon chopped fresh chives

Lobster Salad Sandwich
1 pound cooked lobster meat, roughly chopped
½ cup sliced celery
½ cup finely diced sweet onion
¼ cup finely diced red bell pepper
¼ teaspoon kosher salt

4 whole wheat top-split hot dog buns, lightly toasted
2 cups mesclun

In a medium bowl, combine the yogurt, lemon juice, cayenne, parsley, and chives. Stir in the lobster meat, celery, onion, bell pepper, and salt. Top each of the hot dog buns with greens and divide the lobster salad equally among them.

Yield: 4 servings (1 sandwich each)

Per serving: 255 calories; 29 g protein; 28 g carbohydrates; 4 g fiber; 7 g sugars; 3 g fat; 0.7 g saturated fat; 0 trans fat; 83 mg cholesterol; 789 mg sodium; 175 mg calcium; 0.2 g omega-3 fats; 882 IU vitamin A; 18 mg vitamin C; 2 mg vitamin E; 2 mg iron; 4.5 mg zinc

MANGO, RED ONION, AVOCADO, SPINACH, AND CRAB WRAP

8 ounces cooked lump crabmeat, picked over carefully for shells
½ cup diced mango
¼ cup finely chopped red onion
½ medium avocado, diced
1 tablespoon chopped fresh parsley
2 tablespoons white wine vinegar
2 tablespoons fresh lemon juice
½ teaspoon extra virgin olive oil
½ teaspoon kosher salt
⅛ teaspoon freshly ground black pepper
2 cups baby spinach
4 8-inch whole wheat wraps

In a medium bowl, combine the crab, mango, red onion, avocado, and parsley. In a small bowl, whisk together the vinegar, lemon juice, olive oil, salt, and pepper. Pour over the crab mixture and toss well. Place the spinach and crab mixture down the center of each wrap, fold up the bottom third of the wrap over the mixture, and then fold in each side.

Yield: 4 servings (1 wrap with ½ cup baby spinach and a generous ½ cup crab mixture each)

Per serving: 274 calories; 18 g protein; 30 g carbohydrates; 5 g fiber; 5 g sugars; 7.7 g fat; 0.5 g saturated fat; 0 trans fat; 64 mg cholesterol; 656 mg sodium; 85 mg calcium; 0.04 g omega-3 fats; 699 IU vitamin A; 16 mg vitamin C; 1 mg vitamin E; 2.2 mg iron; 0.2 mg zinc

ROAST BEEF, ARUGULA, AND TOMATO WRAP

4 8-inch whole wheat wraps
¼ cup horseradish mustard
2 cups baby arugula
1 medium tomato, cut into 8 slices
⅓ cup thinly sliced sweet onion
8 ounces thinly sliced roast beef

Spread each wrap with 1 tablespoon mustard and top with ½ cup arugula, 2 slices tomato, a heaping tablespoon of onion, and 2 ounces of roast beef. Roll up and slice in half.

Yield: 4 servings (1 wrap each)

Per serving: 276 calories; 22 g protein; 26 g carbohydrates; 3.5 g fiber; 3 g sugars; 8.5 g fat; 1.4 g saturated fat; 0 trans fat; 32 mg cholesterol; 362 mg sodium; 42 mg calcium; 0.03 g omega-3 fats; 495 IU vitamin A; 8 mg vitamin C; 0.3 mg vitamin E; 3 mg iron; 3 mg zinc

ROASTED CORN, BLACK BEAN, AND TOMATO SALAD

2 ears corn
½ large sweet onion, sliced (about 1 cup)
2 teaspoons extra virgin olive oil
1 teaspoon kosher salt
¼ teaspoon freshly ground black pepper
1 10.5-ounce can black beans, drained and rinsed
1 large tomato (12 ounces), diced
1 lime, juiced (3 tablespoons)
2 teaspoons adobo sauce from canned chipotle in adobo
2 tablespoons chopped fresh cilantro

Preheat the oven to 425°F. Cut the kernels off the ears of corn and toss with the onion, oil, ½ teaspoon of the salt, and the pepper. Roast in the oven until tender and lightly browned, about 15 minutes. Meanwhile, in a large bowl combine the beans, tomato, 2 tablespoons of the lime juice, the adobo sauce, and the remaining ½ teaspoon salt. When the corn is roasted, sprinkle with the remaining 1 tablespoon lime juice as soon as it comes out of the oven and add to the bean and tomato mixture. Stir in the cilantro.

Yield: 4 servings (1¼ cups each)

Per serving: 157 calories; 7 g protein; 28 g carbohydrates; 8 g fiber; 6 g sugars; 3.4 g fat; 0.5 g saturated fat; 0 trans fat; 0 cholesterol; 665 mg sodium; 47 mg calcium; 0.1 g omega-3 fats; 874 IU vitamin A; 21 mg vitamin C; 1 mg vitamin E; 2 mg iron; 1 mg zinc

ROASTED VEGETABLE PITA PIZZA WITH HERBED GOAT CHEESE MEDALLIONS

4 ounces herbed goat cheese
4 portobello mushroom caps, cleaned
1 small red onion, cut into ½-inch-thick rings
2 medium tomatoes, sliced ½ inch thick
1 tablespoon extra virgin olive oil
¼ teaspoon kosher salt
¼ teaspoon freshly ground black pepper
4 whole wheat pitas

Preheat the oven to 400°F. Place the goat cheese in the freezer while you prepare the vegetables, about 20 minutes, for easier slicing. Place the mushroom caps, onion rings, and sliced tomatoes on a baking sheet in a single layer. Drizzle with the oil and season with the salt and pepper. Roast until tender, about 15 minutes. Remove from the oven, but leave the oven on. Remove the goat cheese from the freezer and cut into thin slices. Top each pita equally with the roasted vegetables and goat cheese slices and return to the oven until the cheese is warmed and softened, 3 minutes.

Yield: 4 servings (1 pizza each)

Per serving: 325 calories; 14 g protein; 44 g carbohydrates; 7.2 g fiber; 5 g sugars; 11 g fat; 5 g saturated fat; 0 trans fat; 13 mg cholesterol; 575 mg sodium; 68 mg calcium; 0.1 g omega-3 fats; 914 IU vitamin A; 12 mg vitamin C; 1.3 mg vitamin E; 3.2 mg iron; 2 mg zinc

SALMON CAESAR SALAD WITH TOMATOES AND CREAMY YOGURT DRESSING

Dressing
¼ cup low-fat plain yogurt
1 clove garlic, finely chopped
2 teaspoons fresh lemon juice
¼ teaspoon kosher salt
¼ teaspoon freshly ground black pepper

Salad
1 tablespoon extra virgin olive oil
4 6-ounce wild salmon fillets
8 cups baby spinach
1⅓ cups grape tomatoes
¼ cup coarsely grated Parmesan cheese

In a small bowl, mix together the yogurt, garlic, lemon juice, salt, and pepper. Set aside. Heat the olive oil in a medium nonstick skillet over medium-high heat. Add the salmon fillets, skin side up, and cook until well browned and cooked about halfway through, 5 minutes. Flip and cook until opaque throughout, 8–10 minutes. Remove from the heat and let cool slightly. In a large bowl, combine the baby spinach, grape tomatoes, and half of the dressing. Toss well and divide among 4 plates. Top each with a piece of salmon, drizzle with the remaining dressing, and sprinkle with Parmesan cheese.

Yield: 4 servings (1 salmon filet and generous 1½ cups dressed salad each)

Per serving: 339 calories; 43 g protein; 5.5 g carbohydrates; 2 g fiber; 2.7 g sugars; 15 g fat; 3 g saturated fat; 0 trans fat; 113 mg cholesterol; 452 mg sodium; 160 mg calcium; 3.4 g omega-3 fats; 4,824 IU vitamin A; 21 mg vitamin C; 3.3 mg vitamin E; 3.1 mg iron; 2 mg zinc

SPICY CARROT AND SWEET POTATO SOUP

1 tablespoon extra virgin olive oil
2 cups chopped onion
2 tablespoons chopped garlic
2 tablespoons chopped fresh ginger
2 cinnamon sticks
2 teaspoons cumin seeds, crushed
2 teaspoons coriander seeds, crushed
¼ teaspoon hot red pepper flakes
1 pound carrots, peeled and chopped
2 pounds sweet potatoes, peeled and chopped
2 14.5-ounce cans fat-free chicken broth
3 cups water
3 tablespoons peanut butter
¼ teaspoon kosher salt
⅓ cup chopped fresh cilantro for garnish

In a medium saucepan, heat the olive oil over medium heat and add the onion, garlic, ginger, cinnamon, cumin, coriander, and hot red pepper. Sauté until tender, about 5 minutes, and add the carrots and sweet potatoes. Cook for 5 minutes and add the broth and water. Bring to a simmer and cook until the vegetables are tender, about 25 minutes. Remove from the heat, remove the cinnamon sticks, and, using a hand blender, blend until slightly chunky. Stir in the peanut butter and season with salt. Garnish each bowl with chopped cilantro.

Yield: 4 servings (2 cups each)

Per serving: 331 calories; 9 g protein; 54 g carbohydrates; 10 g fiber; 19.5 g sugars; 10.5 g fat; 1.9 g saturated fat; 0 trans fat; 0 cholesterol; 750 mg sodium; 130 mg calcium; 0.04 g omega-3 fats; 44,855 IU vitamin A; 37 mg vitamin C; 4 mg vitamin E; 3 mg iron; 1.2 mg zinc

SPRING PEA AND SPINACH SOUP WITH CRAB

1 tablespoon extra virgin olive oil
1 onion, chopped
2 cloves garlic, sliced
3 cups fresh or frozen peas
1 14.5-ounce can low-sodium chicken broth
1½ cups water
3 cups baby spinach
½ teaspoon kosher salt
¼ teaspoon freshly ground black pepper
1 cup lump crabmeat, picked over carefully for shells and cartilage
2 teaspoons fresh lemon juice
1 tablespoon finely chopped fresh chives

Heat the oil in a medium saucepan over medium heat. Add the onion and garlic and sauté until the onion is tender and translucent, 5 minutes. Add the peas and sauté for another 2 minutes. Add the broth and water, bring to a simmer, and cook until the peas are tender, 8–10 minutes. Stir in the baby spinach and cook until wilted, 2 minutes. Remove from the heat, puree, and season with ¼ teaspoon of the salt and the pepper. In a small bowl, mix the crabmeat with the remaining ¼ teaspoon salt, the lemon juice, and the chives. Divide the soup among four bowls and top evenly with the crabmeat.

Yield: 4 servings (about 1½ cups soup and ¼ cup crab each)

Per serving: 188 calories; 15 g protein; 22 g carbohydrates; 7 g fiber; 8 g sugars; 5 g fat; 0.8 g saturated fat; 0 trans fat; 29 mg cholesterol; 373 mg sodium; 93 mg calcium; 0.2 g omega-3 fats; 2,505 IU vitamin A; 26 mg vitamin C; 1.5 mg vitamin E; 2.7 mg iron; 3 mg zinc

SWEET AND SPICY CRAB AND KIWI SALAD

8 ounces lump crabmeat, picked over carefully for shells
2 tablespoons fresh lime juice
¼ cup sweet chile sauce
¼ teaspoon kosher salt
¼ teaspoon freshly ground black pepper
1½ cups chopped, peeled kiwi
½ cup finely chopped celery
⅓ cup finely chopped red bell pepper
8 cups mesclun
1 avocado, peeled, pitted, and sliced
⅓ cup toasted sliced almonds

Combine the crab and 1 tablespoon of the lime juice in a small bowl; set aside. In a large bowl, whisk together the remaining 1 tablespoon lime juice, the sweet chile sauce, salt, and pepper. Add the kiwi, celery, bell pepper, and greens. Toss well, divide among 4 plates, and top with the crab, sliced avocado, and almonds.

Yield: 4 servings (2½ cups dressed salad each)

Per serving: 278 calories; 16 g protein; 29 g carbohydrates; 8 g fiber; 13 g sugars; 12 g fat; 1.4 g saturated fat; 0 trans fat; 57 mg cholesterol; 540 mg sodium; 156 mg calcium; 0.4 g omega-3 fats; 1,601 IU vitamin A; 91 mg vitamin C; 5 mg vitamin E; 2 mg iron; 3.5 mg zinc

SWEET POTATO BISQUE WITH SHRIMP

2 tablespoons extra virgin olive oil
12 ounces peeled and deveined extra-large shrimp (19–23 count)
½ teaspoon kosher salt
¼ teaspoon freshly ground black pepper
1 small onion, chopped
1 teaspoon minced garlic
1 pound sweet potatoes, peeled and cubed
1 14.5-ounce can low-sodium chicken broth
2 cups water
2 sprigs fresh thyme
1 cup low-fat plain yogurt

Heat 1 tablespoon of the olive oil in a medium saucepan over medium-high heat. Add the shrimp, season with ¼ teaspoon of the salt and the pepper and sauté until just cooked through, 3–5 minutes. Transfer from the pan to a small bowl and add the remaining 1 tablespoon oil to the pan. Add the onion and garlic and sauté until the onion is translucent and tender, about 3–5 minutes. Add the sweet potatoes and cook until bright orange and slightly softened, about 5 minutes. Add the chicken broth, water, and thyme and bring to a simmer. Cook until the potatoes are very tender, 25–30 minutes. Remove from the heat, discard the thyme sprigs, and puree the soup until smooth. Stir in the yogurt and season with the remaining ¼ teaspoon salt. Top each bowl with shrimp.

Yield: 4 servings (1¼ cups soup and 5 shrimp each)

Per serving: 281 calories; 24 g protein; 24 g carbohydrates; 3 g fiber; 10 g sugars; 10 g fat; 2 g saturated fat; 0 trans fat; 132 mg cholesterol; 462 mg sodium; 182 mg calcium; 0.5 g omega-3 fats; 14,104 IU vitamin A; 15 mg vitamin C; 3 mg vitamin E; 3 mg iron; 2 mg zinc

SWEET POTATO LEEK SOUP

1 tablespoon extra virgin olive oil
1 bunch leeks, trimmed and sliced (2½ cups)
1½ pounds sweet potatoes, peeled and cubed
1 teaspoon fresh thyme leaves, chopped
1 14.5-ounce can low-sodium fat-free chicken broth
1 quart water
¾ teaspoon kosher salt
½ teaspoon freshly ground black pepper
2 tablespoons chopped fresh chives for garnish
¼ cup low-fat plain yogurt for garnish

Heat the oil in a large saucepan until hot but not smoking. Add the leeks and cook until softened, 5 minutes. Add the sweet potatoes and thyme and cook until the sweet potatoes turn bright orange and begin to soften, about 8–10 minutes. Add the broth and water and bring to a simmer. Cook for 20 minutes or until the potatoes are very soft. Remove from the heat and puree with a hand blender. Return to a simmer, season with salt and pepper, and cook until slightly thickened, 5 minutes. Garnish with chives and a dollop of yogurt.

Yield: 4 servings (1½ cups each)

Per serving: 190 calories; 6 g protein; 34 g carbohydrates; 4.5 g fiber; 11 g sugars; 4 g fat; 0.7 g saturated fat; 0 trans fat; 1 mg cholesterol; 582 mg sodium; 109 mg calcium; 0.1 g omega-3 fats; 21,893 IU vitamin A; 25 mg vitamin C; 2.2 mg vitamin E; 2.4 mg iron; 0.5 mg zinc

TURKEY, APPLE, SPINACH, AND CARAMELIZED ONION PRESSED SANDWICH

1 teaspoon extra virgin olive oil
1 large sweet onion, thinly sliced
¼ teaspoon kosher salt
4 cups baby spinach
8 slices whole grain bread
1 pound deli sliced turkey breast
1 apple, thinly sliced
Nonstick cooking spray

Heat the oil in a medium nonstick skillet over medium heat. Add the onion and salt, stir well, and cover. Cook for 5 minutes, uncover, stir, and continue to cook until caramelized, about 10 minutes. Remove from the heat, stir in the spinach until lightly wilted, and place in a small bowl. Wipe out the skillet and set aside. Assemble the sandwiches: top 4 slices of bread with equal amounts of caramelized onions and spinach, turkey, and apple; top with a second slice of bread. Spray a large skillet with nonstick cooking spray set over medium-high heat and cook the sandwiches, pressing down, until golden on each side, 3–4 minutes.

Yield: 4 servings (1 sandwich each)

Per serving: 368 calories; 44 g protein; 37 g carbohydrates; 7 g fiber; 11 g sugars; 4.5 g fat; 0.9 g saturated fat; 0 trans fat; 94 mg cholesterol; 497 mg sodium; 121 mg calcium; 0.1 g omega-3 fats; 2,272 IU vitamin A; 12 mg vitamin C; 1 mg vitamin E; 4 mg iron; 3.3 mg zinc

The Beauty Diet Dinners

ASIAN CITRUS HALIBUT WITH BROWN RICE

Nonstick cooking spray
4 6-ounce skinless halibut fillets
½ teaspoon grated orange zest
½ teaspoon grated lemon zest
½ teaspoon grated lime zest
½ teaspoon kosher salt
¼ teaspoon freshly ground black pepper
2 teaspoons extra virgin olive oil
1 clove garlic, sliced
1 tablespoon chopped fresh ginger
1 tablespoon low-sodium soy sauce
3 tablespoons fresh orange juice
2 tablespoons water
1 scallion, sliced
1 cup brown rice, cooked

Preheat the oven to 425°F and line a baking sheet with aluminum foil sprayed with nonstick cooking spray. Place the halibut, former skin side down, on the baking sheet. In a small dish, combine the three citrus zests with the salt and pepper and mix well. Divide among the halibut fillets, drizzle with the olive oil, and place in the oven. Roast until just cooked through, 10–12 minutes. Meanwhile, combine the garlic, ginger, soy sauce, orange juice, and water in a small skillet and bring to a simmer. Simmer until fragrant and slightly reduced, about 3 minutes. Remove from the heat and stir in scallion. Serve the halibut over the brown rice and top with a drizzle of the soy orange sauce.

Yield: 4 servings (6 ounces halibut, ¾ cup rice, and about 2 tablespoons sauce each)

Per serving: 395 calories; 42 g protein; 37 g carbohydrates; 3 g fiber; 1.5 g sugars; 7.8 g fat; 1.2 g saturated fat; 0 trans fat; 58 mg cholesterol; 439 mg sodium; 107 mg calcium; 0.8 g omega-3 fats; 316 IU vitamin A; 8 mg vitamin C; 2 mg vitamin E; 2.4 mg iron; 2 mg zinc

BRAISED CHICKEN WITH DRIED FRUIT OVER TOASTED WALNUT COUSCOUS

1½ pounds boneless, skinless chicken breasts
½ teaspoon kosher salt
½ teaspoon freshly ground black pepper
1 tablespoon extra virgin olive oil
¼ cup pitted prunes, halved
¼ cup dried apricots, halved
¼ cup fresh orange juice
1 medium red onion, cut into 8 wedges
1 large clove garlic, sliced
1 14.5-ounce can fat-free chicken broth
¼ cup toasted chopped walnuts
3 cups cooked whole wheat couscous
¼ cup fresh parsley leaves, coarsely chopped

Season the chicken with half of the salt and pepper. Heat the olive oil in a deep skillet over medium-high heat and add the chicken breasts. Cook until well browned, about 3–5 minutes, flip, and brown the other side, another 3–5 minutes. Meanwhile, combine the prunes, apricots, and orange juice in a small bowl and microwave for 1½ minutes, until the fruit is softened and about half the liquid has been absorbed. Transfer the browned chicken to a plate, add the onion wedges and garlic to the skillet, and cook until lightly browned and softened, about 5 minutes. Add the plumped fruit and any remaining liquid and stir to scrap up any browned bits from the bottom of the skillet. Add the chicken stock, bring to a simmer, and cook until reduced by one-third. Add the chicken back and cook until it is cooked through and the liquid has reduced to a thickened sauce, 15 minutes. Meanwhile, stir the toasted walnuts into the couscous. When the chicken is cooked and the sauce has reduced, turn off the heat, stir in the parsley, and serve over the walnut couscous.

Yield: 4 servings (6 ounces chicken and ¾ cup couscous each)

Per serving: 442 calories; 46 g protein; 40 g carbohydrates; 6 g fiber; 10 g sugars; 11 g fat; 1.5 g saturated fat; 0 trans fat; 99 mg cholesterol; 582 mg sodium; 56 mg calcium; 0.7 g omega-3 fats; 803 IU vitamin A; 18 mg vitamin C; 1.1 mg vitamin E; 3 mg iron; 2 mg zinc

BROILED OYSTERS FLORENTINE WITH MIXED GREENS

Oysters

24 large oysters, such as bluepoint, shucked
1½ cups cooked chopped spinach, well drained
¼ cup sliced scallion
¾ cup fresh bread crumbs
¼ cup grated Parmesan cheese
¼ teaspoon kosher salt
1½ tablespoons extra virgin olive oil

Salad

8 cups mesclun
1½ cups thinly sliced fennel bulb
1 cup sliced mushrooms
3 tablespoons fresh lemon juice
¼ teaspoon kosher salt
¼ teaspoon freshly ground black pepper
1 tablespoon extra virgin olive oil

Preheat the broiler. Open the oysters and put them in their bottom shells on a baking sheet lined with aluminum foil. In a medium bowl, mix together the spinach, scallion, bread crumbs, Parmesan, and salt and divide evenly among the oysters. Drizzle with olive oil and place under the broiler. Broil for 3–5 minutes or until the oysters are just cooked through and the spinach mixture is lightly browned.

Meanwhile, in a large bowl, toss together the mesclun, fennel, mushrooms, lemon juice, salt, and pepper. Drizzle in the oil and toss again.

Yield: 4 servings (6 oysters and about 2 cups salad each)

Per serving: 234 calories; 12 g protein; 20 g carbohydrates; 5 g fiber; 2 g sugars; 12 g fat; 2.7 g saturated fat; 0 trans fat; 30 mg cholesterol; 642 mg sodium; 270 mg calcium; 0.6 g omega-3 fats; 8,252 IU vitamin A; 29 mg vitamin C; 3.3 mg vitamin E; 10 mg iron; 41 mg zinc

BUTTERMILK SCALLION SMASHED SWEET POTATOES

1 pound sweet potatoes, peeled and cut into 2-inch pieces
1 clove garlic, peeled
½ cup buttermilk
2 scallions, thinly sliced (¼ cup)
¾ teaspoon salt
¼ teaspoon freshly ground black pepper
1 tablespoon butter

Place the potatoes and garlic in a medium saucepan and cover with cold salted water. Bring to a boil, reduce the heat to a simmer, and cook until the potatoes are tender, 15 minutes. Drain well and add the buttermilk, scallions, salt, pepper, and butter. Mash with a fork until just slightly chunky.

Yield: 4 servings (½ cup each)

Per serving: 108 calories; 2.4 g protein; 18 g carbohydrates; 2.4 g fiber; 6.7 g sugars; 3.3 g fat; 2 g saturated fat; 0 trans fat; 9 mg cholesterol; 586 mg sodium; 66 mg calcium; 0.02 g omega-3 fats; 14,080 IU vitamin A; 13 mg vitamin C; 1 mg vitamin E; 1 mg iron; 0.34 mg zinc

EDAMAME SUCCOTASH

1 tablespoon vegetable oil
½ cup diced sweet onion
⅓ cup finely diced red bell pepper
1 jalapeño chile, seeded and diced
1 cup fresh or frozen corn kernels
1½ cups frozen shelled edamame, thawed
¼ cup water
½ teaspoon kosher salt
¼ teaspoon freshly ground pepper
1 teaspoon fresh thyme leaves, chopped

Heat the oil in a medium skillet over medium-high heat; add the onion and sauté until the onion is just beginning to soften, 3 minutes. Add the bell pepper, jalapeño, corn, and edamame. Cook, stirring often, until the peppers are softened and the corn and edamame are softened but still slightly firm, 10 minutes. Add the water, scraping the bottom of the pan, and the salt, pepper, and thyme. Cook until corn and beans are tender throughout and the liquid has cooked off, 5 minutes.

Yield: 4 servings (½ cup each)

Per serving: 218 calories; 14 g protein; 22 g carbohydrates; 6 g fiber; 4 g sugars; 10 g fat; 1 g saturated fat; 0 trans fat; 0 cholesterol; 264 mg sodium; 152 mg calcium; 0.7 g omega-3 fats; 654 IU vitamin A; 39 mg vitamin C; 1 mg vitamin E; 3 mg iron; 1.2 mg zinc

GARLIC HERB LOBSTER TAIL WITH SPINACH AND PEA RISOTTO

5 ounces spinach leaves
1 cup frozen peas, thawed
1 tablespoon butter
1 teaspoon kosher salt
½ teaspoon freshly ground pepper
3 cups water
2 tablespoons extra virgin olive oil
1 small onion, diced
2 large cloves garlic, chopped
¾ cup Arborio rice
⅓ cup white wine
1 14.5-ounce can fat-free chicken stock
2 pounds frozen lobster tails, thawed
2 tablespoons minced fresh herbs, such as rosemary, thyme, and
    parsley
2 tablespoons fresh lemon juice

Bring a large pot of water to a boil and add the spinach leaves. Cook for 1 minute or until deep green and wilted. Drain into a colander and run cold water over the spinach until cool. Squeeze as much liquid as possible out of the spinach and place in a blender. Add the peas, butter, ¼ teaspoon each of the salt and pepper, and as much water as needed to blend into a thick, smooth puree, up to 1 cup. Next, heat 1 tablespoon of the olive oil in a large skillet over medium heat. Add the onion and half of the garlic. Sauté until the onion is translucent and tender, about 5 minutes. Add the rice and continue to cook until the rice is well coated and lightly toasted, about 2 minutes. Carefully add the wine and cook, scraping any brown bits from the bottom of the skillet, until evaporated, about 3–5 minutes. Combine the chicken stock and remaining 2 cups water in a small saucepan and warm. Begin adding the liquid to the rice in ½-cup intervals, making sure all the liquid is evaporated before adding more and stirring constantly. When the rice is tender, stir in the pea puree and season with ½ teaspoon of the remaining salt and the remaining ¼ teaspoon pepper. Set aside. Split the lobster tails and remove the meat in one piece. Heat the remaining 1 tablespoon olive oil in a medium skillet over medium-high heat and add the herbs and remaining clove of garlic. Sauté until fragrant, 1 minute, and then add the lobster. Sauté until just cooked through, 3 minutes, add the lemon juice and remaining ¼ teaspoon salt, and remove from the heat. Serve the lobster over the risotto.

Yield: 4 servings (8 ounces lobster and 1 cup risotto each)

Per serving: 424 calories; 35 g protein; 43 g carbohydrates; 3.4 g fiber; 3.5 g sugars; 12 g fat; 3 g saturated fat; 0 trans fat; 140 mg cholesterol; 1,226 mg sodium; 135 mg calcium; 0.13 g omega-3 fats; 4,333 IU vitamin A; 24 mg vitamin C; 4 mg vitamin E; 3 mg iron; 5 mg zinc

GARLICKY WILTED SPINACH

2 large bunches spinach (about 1¼ pounds, 1 pound trimmed)
½ teaspoon extra virgin olive oil
2 garlic cloves, thinly sliced
⅛ teaspoon kosher salt
⅛ teaspoon freshly ground black pepper

Trim the stems from spinach, wash, and dry well. Heat the oil in a large skillet over medium-high heat. Add the garlic and sauté until fragrant and just turning brown, about 30 seconds. Add the spinach and cook, in batches if necessary, tossing until wilted and bright green, about 2 minutes. Drain any extra liquid from the spinach and season with salt and pepper.

Yield: 4 servings (½ cup each)

GRILLED CHICKEN SKEWERS WITH YOGURT CUCUMBER SAUCE AND CHERRY TOMATO COUSCOUS

1½ pounds boneless, skinless chicken tenderloins
2 cloves garlic, sliced
1 tablespoon extra virgin olive oil
½ teaspoon kosher salt
½ teaspoon freshly ground black pepper
½ cup low-fat plain yogurt
¼ cup finely chopped seedless cucumber
1½ tablespoons white wine vinegar
1 tablespoon chopped fresh parsley
3 cups cooked whole wheat couscous
1 cup halved cherry tomatoes
12 wooden skewers, soaked in water for 30 minutes

Preheat a grill for cooking over direct heat or a grill pan to medium-high heat. Combine the chicken, garlic, oil, and ¼ teaspoon each salt and pepper and marinate for 30 minutes. Meanwhile, in a small bowl, mix the yogurt, cucumber, vinegar, parsley, and remaining ¼ teaspoon each salt and pepper. Fluff the couscous with a fork and stir in the cherry tomatoes. Thread the chicken on the skewers and grill until just cooked through, 4–6 minutes on each side. Serve over the couscous with yogurt sauce on the side.

Yield: 4 servings (3 chicken skewers, 1 cup couscous, and about 3 tablespoons sauce each)

GRILLED HALIBUT AND VEGETABLE SKEWERS

2 tablespoons extra virgin olive oil
2 cloves garlic, sliced
½ teaspoon hot red pepper flakes
12 white mushrooms, halved
1 small onion, cut into 8 wedges
1 green bell pepper, cut into 12 pieces
1 cup cherry tomatoes
½ teaspoon kosher salt
12 wooden skewers, soaked in water for 30 minutes
1½ pounds halibut, skin removed and cut into 2- to 3-inch pieces
Lemon wedges, for garnish

Preheat a grill or grill pan over medium-high heat. Heat the oil in a small saucepan over medium heat with the garlic and red pepper flakes until the garlic is just golden, about 1–2 minutes. Remove from the heat and let cool. Place the mushrooms, onion, bell pepper, and cherry tomatoes in a medium bowl. Toss with half the flavored oil and ¼ teaspoon of the salt. Thread onto 8 skewers. Place the halibut in the same bowl and toss with the remaining oil and remaining ¼ teaspoon salt. Thread onto the remaining 4 skewers. Grill until the halibut is just cooked through and the vegetables are crisp-tender, 4–5 minutes on each side. Serve with fresh lemon wedges on the side.

Yield: 4 servings (6 ounces halibut and 2 vegetable skewers each)

Per serving: 340 calories; 49 g protein; 8 g carbohydrates; 2 g fiber; 4 g sugars; 12 g fat; 1.8 g saturated fat; 0 trans fat; 70 mg cholesterol; 366 mg sodium; 119 mg calcium; 1 g omega-3 fats; 847 IU vitamin A; 38 mg vitamin C; 3 mg vitamin E; 2.5 mg iron; 1.4 mg zinc

GRILLED SALMON WITH MANGO KIWI SALSA

Nonstick cooking spray
4 6-ounce wild salmon fillets
½ teaspoon cumin seeds, crushed
¼ to ½ teaspoon chipotle powder
1 teaspoon kosher salt

1 ripe mango, peeled and cut into small cubes
4 kiwis, peeled and cut into small cubes
1 small red onion, sliced thin
Juice of 1 lime
½ teaspoon freshly ground black pepper
¼ cup cilantro leaves, finely chopped

Preheat a grill for direct heat cooking or a nonstick grill pan sprayed with nonstick cooking spray over medium-high heat. Season the salmon fillets with the cumin, chipotle, and half of the salt. Place skin side up on the grill pan and cook until well marked, 5–7 minutes. Flip and continue to grill until just cooked through. Meanwhile, combine the mango, kiwis, red onion, lime juice, pepper, cilantro, and remaining ½ teaspoon salt and toss well to combine. Set aside until the salmon is ready. Serve the salsa over the salmon.

Yield: 4 servings (6 ounces salmon and about ½ cup salsa each)

Per serving: 369 calories; 40 g protein; 23 g carbohydrates; 4 g fiber; 15 g sugars; 13 g fat; 2 g saturated fat; 0 trans fat; 107 mg cholesterol; 572 mg sodium; 65 mg calcium; 3.4 g omega-3 fats; 656 IU vitamin A; 90 mg vitamin C; 4 mg vitamin E; 2.2 mg iron; 1.4 mg zinc

GRILLED STRIPED BASS WITH LEMONY SPINACH AND SUGAR SNAP PEA SAUTÉ

4 6-ounce striped bass fillets
½ teaspoon kosher salt
½ teaspoon freshly ground black pepper
1 teaspoon grated lemon zest
1 tablespoon extra virgin olive oil
1 pound sugar snap peas, trimmed
4 cups baby spinach
1 tablespoon fresh lemon juice, plus lemon wedges for garnish

Preheat a grill for cooking over direct heat or heat a grill pan over medium-high heat. Season the bass fillets with ¼ teaspoon each of the salt and pepper and the lemon zest. Grill until just cooked through and flaky, 4 to 5 minutes on each side. Meanwhile, heat the olive oil in a medium skillet over medium heat and add the sugar snap peas. Sauté until crisp-tender, 5 minutes. Add the spinach and continue to cook until wilted, 2 to 3 minutes. Season with the remaining ¼ teaspoon each salt and pepper and the fresh lemon juice. Serve the bass over the peas and spinach with lemon wedges for garnish.

Yield: 4 servings (6 ounces bass and ¾ cup snap peas and spinach each)

Per serving: 261 calories; 34 g protein; 11 g carbohydrates; 3.3 g fiber; 4 g sugars; 7.7 g fat; 1 g saturated fat; 0 trans fat; 140 mg cholesterol; 393 mg sodium; 132 mg calcium; 1.4 g omega-3 fats; 3,394 IU vitamin A; 29 mg vitamin C; 2 mg vitamin E; 3.6 mg iron; 1 mg zinc

GRILLED SWEET POTATO "FRIES"

Nonstick cooking spray
1½ pounds sweet potatoes, scrubbed
1 teaspoon extra virgin olive oil
¾ teaspoon kosher salt
¼ teaspoon hot red pepper flakes

Preheat a nonstick grill pan sprayed with nonstick cooking spray over medium heat. Cut the potatoes into thick wedges (each one should weigh about an ounce, and you should have about 24) and toss in a bowl with the oil, salt, and hot red pepper. Place on the grill and cover with the lid of a pot or aluminum foil. Cook for 8–10 minutes on each side or until tender.

Yield: 4 servings (about 6 potato wedges each)

Per serving: 143 calories; 3 g protein; 30 g carbohydrates; 5.3 g fiber; 9 g sugars; 1 g fat; 0 saturated fat; 0 trans fat; 0 cholesterol; 453 mg sodium; 27 mg calcium; 0.01 g omega-3 fats; 7,897 IU vitamin A; 24 mg vitamin C; 0.2 mg vitamin E; 1 mg iron; 0 zinc

GRILLED TURKEY CUTLETS WITH SWEET AND SPICY BLUEBERRY CRANBERRY RELISH

Nonstick cooking spray
1½ pounds turkey cutlets
½ teaspoon kosher salt
¼ teaspoon freshly ground black pepper
½ cup cranberries
2 tablespoons sugar
½ chipotle chile canned in adobo sauce
1 scallion, chopped
½ cup blueberries

Preheat a grill or grill pan sprayed with nonstick cooking spray over medium-high heat. Season the turkey with ¼ teaspoon of the salt and the pepper and place on the grill; grill for about 5 minutes on each side or until just cooked through and no longer pink. Meanwhile, in a food processor, pulse the remaining ¼ teaspoon salt, the cranberries, sugar, and chipotle until finely ground and well mixed. Add the scallion and blueberries and pulse 3–5 times or until incorporated but still chunky. Serve over the turkey.

Yield: 4 servings (6 ounces turkey and 2 tablespoons relish each)

Per serving: 224 calories; 41 g protein; 11 g carbohydrates; 1.2 g fiber; 8.7 g sugars; 1.2 g fat; 0.3 g saturated fat; 0 trans fat; 111 mg cholesterol; 316 mg sodium; 23 mg calcium; 0.03 g omega-3 fats; 77 IU vitamin A; 4.2 mg vitamin C; 0.4 mg vitamin E; 2.3 mg iron; 2.4 mg zinc

HERB-BAKED SALMON WITH WARM CHERRY TOMATO SALAD AND WHOLE WHEAT COUSCOUS

Salmon
4 6-ounce wild salmon fillets
2 cloves garlic, minced
3 tablespoons chopped mixed fresh herbs, such as rosemary, thyme, and basil
1 teaspoon extra virgin olive oil
1 teaspoon kosher salt
½ teaspoon freshly ground black pepper

Tomato Salad and Couscous

1 teaspoon extra virgin olive oil
1 clove garlic, sliced
2 scallions, cut into 1-inch pieces (¼ cup)
2 cups grape or cherry tomatoes, halved
¼ teaspoon kosher salt
¼ teaspoon freshly ground black pepper
1 teaspoon apple cider vinegar
3 cups cooked whole wheat couscous

Preheat the oven to 400°F. Place the salmon, skin side down, on a foil-lined baking sheet. Using a sharp knife, make two slits, each about 3 inches long, across the fattest part of the fillets. Combine the garlic, herbs, and olive oil in a small bowl and stuff about 1 teaspoon of this mixture into each slit. Season the fillets with salt and pepper and bake until just cooked through, 8–10 minutes.

Meanwhile, for the tomato salad, heat the oil in a medium skillet over medium-high heat. Add the garlic and scallions and cook until slightly softened and lightly browned, about 2 minutes. Add the tomatoes, salt, and pepper and cook for 1 minute, until the tomatoes are warmed. Stir in the vinegar and set aside.

To serve, divide the cooked couscous among four plates and top with the tomato salad and a fillet of salmon.

Note: When removing salmon from the aluminum foil, place the spatula just above the skin of the salmon and slide it in. This will allow you to lift the salmon off the aluminum foil and leave the skin behind.

Yield: 4 servings (¾ cup couscous, ½ cup tomato salad, and one 6-ounce salmon fillet each)

Per serving: 423 calories; 44 g protein; 27 g carbohydrates; 5 g fiber; 2 g sugars; 15 g fat; 2 g saturated fat; 0 trans fat; 107 mg cholesterol; 693 mg sodium; 56 mg calcium; 3.4 g omega-3 fats; 829 IU vitamin A; 13 mg vitamin C; 3 mg vitamin E; 3 mg iron; 1.5 mg zinc

LEMONY ROASTED CHICKEN AND ARTICHOKES

1 lemon
4 artichokes, trimmed to the heart and halved
4 garlic cloves, crushed
2 sprigs fresh rosemary, plus 1 tablespoon chopped
1 tablespoon extra virgin olive oil
½ teaspoon kosher salt
½ teaspoon freshly ground black pepper
1½ pounds boneless, skinless chicken breast

Preheat the oven to 450°F. Line a baking sheet with foil and set aside.

Fill a large saucepan with water. Squeeze the lemon into the water. Add the artichokes, garlic, and rosemary sprigs and bring to a boil. Cook until the artichokes are just tender when pierced with a knife, about 10 minutes. Drain and place on the baking sheet. Toss with 2 teaspoons of the oil and ¼ teaspoon each of the salt and pepper. Push to one side of the baking sheet. Place the chicken breasts on the other side of the baking sheet and season with the remaining salt and pepper and the chopped rosemary. Drizzle with the remaining 1 teaspoon olive oil and place in the oven. Roast for 15 minutes or until the chicken is just cooked through and the artichokes are browned and softened.

Yield: 4 servings (6 ounces chicken and 2 artichoke halves each)

Per serving: 244 calories; 36 g protein; 7 g carbohydrates; 3.2 g fiber; 0.6 g sugars; 7.5 g fat; 1.7 g saturated fat; 0 trans fat; 94 mg cholesterol; 377 mg sodium; 45 mg calcium; 0.1 g omega-3 fats; 139 IU vitamin A; 6 mg vitamin C; 1 mg vitamin E; 2 mg iron; 1.4 mg zinc

MUSTARD-CRUSTED SALMON WITH ROASTED GREEN BEANS AND SHALLOTS

Nonstick cooking spray
1 pound green beans, trimmed
2 shallots, sliced
2 teaspoons extra virgin olive oil
½ teaspoon kosher salt
½ teaspoon freshly ground black pepper
4 6-ounce wild salmon fillets
2 tablespoons Dijon mustard
2 teaspoons honey

Preheat the oven to 425°F. Line a baking sheet with foil and spray with nonstick cooking spray; set aside. Bring a large pot of water to a boil, add the green beans, and boil for 3–5 minutes or until bright green and slightly tender. Drain and run under cold water until cool. Drain well; toss with the shallots, oil, salt, and ¼ teaspoon of the pepper; and place on one half of the baking sheet. Place the salmon fillets, skin side down, on the other half of the baking sheet. In a small bowl, mix the mustard and honey and spread evenly on the salmon fillets. Season with the remaining ¼ teaspoon pepper and roast in the oven until the salmon is just cooked through and the beans are lightly browned, 12–14 minutes.

Yield: 4 servings (6 ounces salmon and 4 ounces green beans each)

Per serving: 365 calories; 41 g protein; 16 g carbohydrates; 4 g fiber; 5 g sugars; 15 g fat; 2 g saturated fat; 0 trans fat; 107 mg cholesterol; 516 mg sodium; 79 mg calcium; 3.5 g omega-3 fats; 1,024 IU vitamin A; 12 mg vitamin C; 3 mg vitamin E; 2.6 mg iron; 1.6 mg zinc

OVEN-CRUNCHY WALNUT CHICKEN TENDERS

Nonstick cooking spray
1½ pounds chicken tenderloins
2 tablespoons buttermilk
½ teaspoon salt
1 cup panko
¼ cup finely chopped walnuts

Preheat the oven to 450°F. Line a baking sheet with foil and spray with nonstick cooking spray. In a medium bowl, toss the chicken with the buttermilk and salt. Let sit for 10 minutes. Sprinkle the panko and walnuts directly into the bowl and toss well, coating all the tenders. Place on the prepared baking sheet and bake for 15 minutes or until the chicken is just cooked through and the crumbs are golden.

Yield: 4 servings (6 ounces chicken each)

Per serving: 290 calories; 37 g protein; 12 g carbohydrates; 1.1 g fiber; 1 g sugars; 9.5 g fat; 1.8 g saturated fat; 0 trans fat; 94 mg cholesterol; 422 mg sodium; 37 mg calcium; 0.73 g omega-3 fats; 26 IU vitamin A; 0.3 mg vitamin C; 0.4 mg vitamin E; 1.5 mg iron; 1.4 mg zinc

OYSTERS ON THE HALF SHELL WITH FRESH TOMATO MIGNONETTE, MIXED GREEN SALAD, AND WHOLE WHEAT BAGUETTE

1 medium tomato, peeled and finely diced
2 tablespoons red wine vinegar
1 tablespoon minced shallot
½ teaspoon cracked black pepper
6 cups baby spinach
1 Belgian endive, sliced into thin rounds
1 radicchio, halved and sliced
1 tablespoon honey
3 tablespoons balsamic vinegar
¼ teaspoon kosher salt
2 tablespoons extra virgin olive oil
24 oysters on the half shell
1 12-ounce whole wheat baguette

In a medium bowl, combine the tomato, red wine vinegar, shallot, and ¼ teaspoon of the cracked black pepper. Let sit at room temperature for about 15 minutes for the flavors to mingle while you prepare the salad. In a large bowl, combine the baby spinach, endive, and radicchio. Whisk the honey, basalmic vinegar, remaining ¼ teaspoon cracked black pepper, and salt until combined and then drizzle in the oil until incorporated; toss with the salad. Divide the tomato mignonette among the oysters and serve with the salad and baguette.

Yield: 4 servings (6 oysters, 2 cups dressed salad, and 3 ounces baguette each)

Per serving: 374 calories; 15 g protein; 55 g carbohydrates; 7.4 g fiber; 16 g sugars; 12 g fat; 2 g saturated fat; 0 trans fat; 21 mg cholesterol; 723 mg sodium; 166 mg calcium; 0.5 g omega-3 fats; 3,770 IU vitamin A; 21 mg vitamin C; 3 mg vitamin E; 9.3 mg iron; 33 mg zinc

OYSTERS PRIMAVERA

1 head broccoli, cut into small florets (3 cups)
½ cup water
1 small red onion, chopped
1 red bell pepper, sliced
1 small yellow squash, sliced
⅓ cup dry white wine
2 cloves garlic, chopped
16 oysters, shucked
¼ teaspoon kosher salt
¼ teaspoon freshly ground black pepper
½ teaspoon grated lemon zest
¼ cup fresh parsley leaves, chopped
3 cups cooked brown rice

Place the broccoli and water in a large sauté pan. Bring to a boil and cook until the broccoli is bright green and slightly tender, about 5 minutes. Add the onion, bell pepper, and squash and continue to sauté until the vegetables are crisp-tender, 5–7 minutes. Add the wine, garlic, and oysters and cook for 3–5 minutes or until the oysters are just cooked through. Remove from the heat and season with salt, pepper, and lemon zest. Stir the parsley into the cooked brown rice and serve under the oysters primavera.

Yield: 4 servings (about 1½ cups oysters primavera and ¾ cup rice each)

Per serving: 245 calories; 9 g protein; 47 g carbohydrates; 6 g fiber; 4 g sugars; 2.5 g fat; 0.5 g saturated fat; 0 trans fat; 14 mg cholesterol; 243 mg sodium; 88 mg calcium; 0.4 g omega-3 fats; 3,154 IU vitamin A; 113 mg vitamin C; 1.6 mg vitamin E; 5 mg iron; 22.6 mg zinc

PINEAPPLE- AND RUM-MARINATED GRILLED CHICKEN OVER GRILLED SWEET POTATO SALAD

1½ pounds chicken tenderloins
¼ cup light or white rum
¼ cup pineapple juice
¼ cup fresh cilantro leaves, plus 2 tablespoons chopped
¾ teaspoon kosher salt

½ teaspoon freshly ground black pepper
1½ pounds sweet potatoes, sliced into ¼ inch rounds
2 tablespoons extra virgin olive oil
2 tablespoons white wine vinegar

Preheat a grill for cooking over direct heat or preheat a grill pan over medium heat. Place the chicken in a resealable plastic bag and add the rum, pineapple juice, ¼ cup cilantro leaves, and ¼ teaspoon each of the salt and pepper. Marinate in the refrigerator for 1 hour. Meanwhile, toss the sweet potato slices with 1 tablespoon of the oil, ¼ teaspoon of the remaining salt, and the remaining ¼ teaspoon pepper. Place on the grill and cover. Cook for 8 to 10 minutes on each side or until cooked through and well marked. Place in a medium bowl and add the remaining 1 tablespoon oil, the vinegar, and the chopped cilantro. Set aside. Remove the chicken from the marinade, pat dry, season with the remaining ¼ teaspoon salt, and place on the grill. Grill until just cooked through, 5 minutes on each side. Serve over the sweet potato salad.

Yield: 4 servings (about 3–4 pieces tenderloin and ¾ cup potato salad each)

Per serving: 340 calories; 36 g protein; 22 g carbohydrates; 3.4 g fiber; 7 g sugars; 11 g fat; 2 g saturated fat; 0 trans fat; 94 mg cholesterol; 420 mg sodium; 57 mg calcium; 0.1 g omega-3 fats; 19,960 IU vitamin A; 21 mg vitamin C; 2 mg vitamin E; 2 mg iron; 1.4 mg zinc

POACHED OYSTERS IN GARLIC, HERBS, AND BROTH WITH MIXED GREENS AND WHOLE WHEAT BAGUETTE

2 teaspoons extra virgin olive oil
2 tablespoons chopped garlic
1 14.5-ounce can fat-free chicken broth
½ cup packed fresh parsley leaves, chopped
2 teaspoons fresh thyme leaves, chopped
½ teaspoon freshly ground black pepper
24 large oysters, such as bluepoint, shucked
6 cups mesclun
2 tablespoons balsamic vinegar
¼ teaspoon kosher salt
1 medium whole wheat baguette (about 12 ounces)

Heat 1 teaspoon of the olive oil in a medium saucepan over medium-high heat. Add the garlic and cook until fragrant and just turning brown, 1 minute. Add the broth and cook until reduced by half, about 8–10 minutes. Reduce the heat to produce a low simmer. Add the herbs, pepper, and oysters and cook for 1 minute. Remove from the heat.

Place the mesclun in a medium bowl and toss with the vinegar, remaining olive oil, and salt. Serve with the oysters, their broth, and whole wheat baguette.

Yield: 4 servings (6 oysters, 1½ cups mesclun, and 3 ounces baguette each)

Per serving: 325 calories; 16 g protein; 50 g carbohydrates; 7 g fiber; 10 g sugars; 7.3 g fat; 1.5 g saturated fat; 0 trans fat; 26 mg cholesterol; 964 mg sodium; 178 mg calcium; 0.5 g omega-3 fats; 1,443 IU vitamin A; 22.5 mg vitamin C; 1.4 mg vitamin E; 10 mg iron; 41 mg zinc

ROASTED BROCCOLI

2 large heads broccoli, trimmed into florets (6 cups/1 pound)
3 cloves garlic, sliced
1 tablespoon extra virgin olive oil
½ teaspoon kosher salt
½ teaspoon freshly ground black pepper
½ teaspoon grated lemon zest

Preheat the oven to 400°F. In a medium bowl, toss together the broccoli, garlic, oil, salt, and pepper. Spread in a single layer on a baking sheet and roast for 15 minutes, or until tender and lightly browned. Remove from the oven and toss with the lemon zest while still warm.

Yield: 4 servings (1 cup each)

Per serving: 65 calories; 3.4 g protein; 6.5 g carbohydrates; 3.2 g fiber; 0 sugars; 4 g fat; 0.5 g saturated fat; 0 trans fat; 0 cholesterol; 270 mg sodium; 57 mg calcium; 0.2 g omega-3 fats; 3,196 IU vitamin A; 100 mg vitamin C; 1 mg vitamin E; 1 mg iron; 0.5 mg zinc

ROSEMARY-ROASTED CHICKEN AND LEEKS WITH SLOW-ROASTED TOMATOES

4 plum tomatoes, cored and sliced thick
2 tablespoons extra virgin olive oil
1 teaspoon fresh thyme leaves
¾ teaspoon kosher salt
½ teaspoon freshly ground black pepper
1 bunch leeks, halved lengthwise, sliced, and rinsed well
1 teaspoon chopped fresh rosemary, plus 1 whole sprig
1½ pounds boneless, skinless chicken breasts

Preheat the oven to 300°F. Line a small baking sheet with parchment paper and spread the tomato slices on it in a single layer. Season with 1 tablespoon of the oil, the thyme leaves, and ¼ teaspoon each of the salt and pepper. Bake for 30 minutes, or until the tomatoes are very soft and have released their juices. Leave them in the oven and turn the temperature up to 425°F. Heat the remaining oil in a large ovenproof skillet and add the leeks. Season them with ¼ teaspoon of the remaining salt and add the whole rosemary sprig. Sauté until the leeks have reduced by half in volume and are slightly softened, 5 minutes. Remove from the heat and place the chicken breasts on top of the leeks. Season the chicken with the remaining ¼ teaspoon each salt and pepper and the chopped rosemary. Place in the oven and roast until the chicken is just cooked through, 12–15 minutes. Remove the tomatoes and chicken from the oven and let stand for 5 minutes. Remove the rosemary sprig from the leeks. Slice the chicken and serve with the leeks and tomatoes.

Yield: 4 servings (6 ounces chicken, about ½ cup leeks, and 3–4 tomato slices each)

Per serving: 301 calories; 41 g protein; 12 g carbohydrates; 2 g fiber; 3 g sugars; 9.5 g fat; 1.6 g saturated fat; 0 trans fat; 98 mg cholesterol; 488 mg sodium; 65 mg calcium; 0.2 g omega-3 fats; 625 IU vitamin A; 16 mg vitamin C; 2.2 mg vitamin E; 3 mg iron; 1.6 mg zinc

SAUTÉED MEDITERRANEAN SHRIMP, TOMATOES, AND BROCCOLI OVER WHOLE WHEAT SPAGHETTI

1 pound peeled and deveined jumbo shrimp (21–25 count)
¼ cup fresh lemon juice
1 tablespoon chopped garlic
½ teaspoon kosher salt
½ teaspoon freshly ground black pepper
2 tablespoons fresh oregano, chopped
1 tablespoon fresh thyme leaves
1 tablespoon extra virgin olive oil
1 large head broccoli, trimmed into florets (3½ cups)
¼ cup water
½ large onion, thinly sliced (1½ cups)
1 cup halved cherry tomatoes
1 pound whole wheat spaghetti, cooked according to package
    directions

Combine the shrimp, 2 tablespoons of the lemon juice, 1 teaspoon of the garlic, ¼ teaspoon each of the salt and pepper, 1 tablespoon of the oregano, 1 teaspoon of the thyme, and 1 teaspoon of the olive oil in a medium bowl. Set aside to marinate.

Place the broccoli and water in a large skillet. Bring to a boil, cover, and simmer for 5 minutes, until bright green and just beginning to soften. Uncover and cook until the remaining water has evaporated. Add the onion, remaining garlic, and remaining salt and pepper and sauté until tender, about 5 minutes. Add the tomatoes and remaining oregano and thyme and cook until just softened, 2 minutes. Remove from the pan and set aside. Heat the remaining 2 teaspoons of olive oil in the same skillet over medium-high heat, add the shrimp and marinade, and sauté until just cooked through, about 3–5 minutes. Add the vegetable mixture to the shrimp, toss to combine, season with the remaining 2 tablespoons lemon juice, and serve over the spaghetti.

Yield: 4 servings (1½ cups shrimp mixture and 4 ounces pasta)

Per serving: 344 calories; 32 g protein; 42.5 g carbohydrates; 8.3 g fiber; 4 g sugars; 6.5 g fat; 1 g saturated fat; 0 trans fat; 172 mg cholesterol; 433 mg sodium; 138 mg calcium; 0.7 g omega-3 fats; 2,455 IU vitamin A; 78 mg vitamin C; 2.5 mg vitamin E; 5 mg iron; 3 mg zinc

SEARED TUNA OVER CONFETTI GLASS NOODLE SALAD

4 ounces cellophane noodles
1 tablespoon extra virgin olive oil
½ cup finely chopped red bell pepper
1 cup finely chopped zucchini
1 small carrot, shredded
1 small onion, halved and sliced lengthwise
2 cups baby spinach, roughly chopped
¾ teaspoon kosher salt
1 teaspoon dark toasted sesame oil
Nonstick cooking spray
4 8-ounce tuna steaks, 1½ inches thick
¼ teaspoon freshly ground black pepper
2 teaspoons sesame seeds

Place the cellophane noodles in a large bowl and cover with boiling water. Let sit until softened, 3–5 minutes, drain well, and cut into 6-inch pieces with kitchen shears; set aside. Heat the olive oil in a medium sauté pan over medium-high heat until hot but not smoking. Add the bell pepper, zucchini, carrot, and onion and sauté until crisp-tender, 3–5 minutes. Add the noodles, toss well, and turn off the heat. Add the spinach, ¼ teaspoon of the salt, and the sesame oil and toss until the spinach is wilted and all the vegetables are well incorporated; set aside. Heat a large nonstick skillet sprayed with nonstick cooking spray. Season the tuna steaks on both sides with the remaining ½ teaspoon salt, the pepper, and the sesame seeds and add to the pan. Sear for 3 minutes on each side and serve over the noodles.

Yield: 4 servings (1 tuna steak and about 1¼ cups noodle mixture each)

Per serving: 420 calories; 54 g protein; 30 g carbohydrates; 2 g fiber; 2.5 g sugars; 8 g fat; 1 g saturated fat; 0 trans fat; 102 mg cholesterol; 469 mg sodium; 85 mg calcium; 0.6 g omega-3 fats; 4,074 IU vitamin A; 34 mg vitamin C; 2.3 mg vitamin E; 3 mg iron; 2 mg zinc

SHRIMP AND ANGEL HAIR PASTA WITH BABY SPINACH AND SLICED MUSHROOM SALAD

Pasta
8 ounces dried angel hair pasta
1 pound peeled and deveined jumbo shrimp (21–25 count)
4 cloves garlic, sliced
½ teaspoon kosher salt
½ teaspoon freshly ground black pepper
1 tablespoon extra virgin olive oil
1 pound ripe tomatoes, diced
¼ cup fresh basil leaves, chopped
1 tablespoon white wine vinegar

Salad
6 cups baby spinach
1½ cups sliced white mushrooms
2 tablespoons fresh lemon juice
1 tablespoon extra virgin olive oil
¼ teaspoon kosher salt
¼ teaspoon freshly ground black pepper

Bring a large pot of water to a boil, add the pasta, and cook according to the package directions. Drain and keep warm. In a medium bowl, combine the shrimp, half of the garlic, and ¼ teaspoon each of the salt and pepper and toss well. Heat the oil in a medium skillet until hot but not smoking and add the shrimp mixture. Cook, stirring, until the shrimp are just cooked through, 3 minutes; transfer to a bowl. Add the tomatoes and remaining garlic to the skillet and cook until the tomatoes soften and release some of their juices, 5 minutes. Add the shrimp back to the pan; add the basil, vinegar, and remaining ¼ teaspoon each salt and pepper; and turn off the heat. Toss well with the cooked pasta.

Combine the spinach and mushrooms in a large bowl and toss with the lemon juice. Add the oil, salt, and pepper and toss again until combined.

Yield: 4 servings (1½ generous cups pasta and 1½ cups salad each)

Per serving: 427 calories; 34 g protein; 50 g carbohydrates; 4.4 g fiber; 5 g sugars; 9.5 g fat; 1.5 g saturated fat; 0 trans fat; 221 mg cholesterol; 656 mg sodium; 117 mg calcium; 0.5 g omega-3 fats; 4,774 IU vitamin A; 32 mg vitamin C; 4 mg vitamin E; 7 mg iron; 3.2 mg zinc

SHRIMP, SWEET POTATO, AND VEGETABLE CURRY OVER COCONUT-LIME JASMINE RICE

1 tablespoon canola oil
2 cloves garlic, thinly sliced
1 2-inch piece fresh ginger, peeled and cut into strips
1 tablespoon red curry paste
1 small sweet onion, sliced
1 medium sweet potato, peeled and cubed (2 cups)
1 red bell pepper, sliced
1 14-ounce can light coconut milk
1½ cups green beans, trimmed and cut into 2-inch pieces
1 pound peeled and deveined jumbo shrimp (21–25 count)
1 tablespoon low-sodium soy sauce
3 tablespoons freshly squeezed lime juice, plus 1 lime, cut into wedges
½ teaspoon kosher salt
½ cup fresh basil leaves, roughly chopped
½ cup fresh cilantro leaves, roughly chopped
1 cup jasmine rice, cooked
½ teaspoon finely grated lime zest
¼ cup toasted sweetened flaked coconut

Heat the oil in a large deep skillet or saucepan over medium-high heat; add the garlic and ginger and sauté until fragrant and just beginning to brown, 1 minute. Add the curry paste and continue to sauté until well incorporated and fragrant, 1 minute, and then quickly stir in the onion, sweet potato, and red bell pepper until coated with curry paste. Add the coconut milk, bring to a simmer, and cook until the sweet potato is tender, about 10 minutes. Add the green beans and shrimp and continue to simmer until the beans are tender and the shrimp have cooked through, 5 minutes. Season with soy sauce, lime juice, and salt; remove from the heat; and stir in the basil and cilantro. In a medium bowl, combine the hot cooked rice, lime zest, and toasted coconut until mixed well. Serve the curry over the rice with extra lime wedges on the side.

Yield: 4 servings (about 1½ cups curry and ¾ cup rice each)

Per serving: 469 calories; 25 g protein; 59 g carbohydrates; 6 g fiber; 11 g sugars; 15 g fat; 6.8 g saturated fat; 0 trans fat; 168 mg cholesterol; 640 mg sodium; 143 mg calcium; 0.7 g omega-3 fats; 8,014 IU vitamin A; 72 mg vitamin C; 3 mg vitamin E; 7.2 mg iron; 2.4 mg zinc

SMOKY SHRIMP FAJITAS WITH WHOLE WHEAT TORTILLAS

1 pound peeled and deveined extra-large shrimp (26–30 count)
2 cloves garlic, sliced
1 tablespoon adobo sauce from canned chipotle in adobo
1 teaspoon honey
1 tablespoon extra virgin olive oil
¼ teaspoon ground cumin
1 small onion, sliced
1 red bell pepper, sliced
1 yellow bell pepper, sliced
½ teaspoon kosher salt
3 tablespoons chopped fresh cilantro
1 tablespoon fresh lime juice
¼ cup low-fat plain yogurt
¼ cup chopped tomato
4 8-inch whole wheat tortillas, warmed

In a medium bowl, combine the shrimp, garlic, adobo sauce, and honey. Toss well and let sit for 10 minutes. Heat the olive oil in a medium skillet over medium-high heat and add the shrimp. Sauté until just cooked through, 3–5 minutes. Transfer from the skillet to a small bowl and add the cumin, onion, bell peppers, and salt. Sauté until crisp-tender, 5 minutes. Add the shrimp back to the vegetables, add 2 tablespoons of the chopped cilantro and the lime juice, and toss well. Meanwhile, in a small bowl, stir together the yogurt, tomato, and remaining 1 tablespoon chopped cilantro. Top each warmed tortilla with the shrimp mixture and yogurt sauce.

Yield: 4 servings (1 fajita each)

Per serving: 342 calories; 29 g protein; 33 g carbohydrates; 3.4 g fiber; 7 g sugars; 9 g fat; 1 g saturated fat; 0 trans fat; 173 mg cholesterol; 602 mg sodium; 107 mg calcium; 0.6 g omega-3 fats; 2,444 IU vitamin A; 137 mg vitamin C; 2.6 mg vitamin E; 4.4 mg iron; 1.6 mg zinc

SPICED SALMON

1 teaspoon jerk seasoning
½ teaspoon kosher salt
⅛ teaspoon chipotle powder
4 6-ounce wild salmon fillets
1½ teaspoons extra virgin olive oil

Preheat the oven to 425°F and line a baking sheet with foil; set aside. In a small bowl, combine the jerk seasoning, salt, and chipotle powder. Season the flesh side of the fillets evenly with this mixture. Heat the olive oil in a large skillet over medium-high heat until hot but not smoking and carefully place the fillets, seasoned side down, in the hot oil. Cook, without moving, until well browned, about 3 minutes. Remove the fillets from the skillet and place on the baking sheet, skin side down. Place in the oven and roast until just cooked through, 6–8 minutes.

Yield: 4 servings (1 filet each)

Per serving: 291 calories; 38.5 g protein; 0 carbohydrates; 0 fiber; 0 sugars; 14 g fat; 2 g saturated fat; 0 trans fat; 107 mg cholesterol; 396 mg sodium; 23 mg calcium; 3.4 g omega-3 fats; 67 IU vitamin A; 0 vitamin C; 2 mg vitamin E; 1.6 mg iron; 1.2 mg zinc

SWEET AND CRUNCHY SHRIMP–SPINACH SALAD

1 pound peeled and deveined jumbo shrimp (21–25 count)
1 egg white, lightly beaten
¼ teaspoon kosher salt
¼ teaspoon freshly ground black pepper
½ cup panko
2 tablespoons extra virgin olive oil
2 tablespoons maple syrup
8 cups baby spinach
⅓ cup thinly sliced red onion
¼ cup toasted chopped walnuts
1 tablespoon white wine vinegar

In a medium bowl, combine the shrimp, beaten egg white, salt, and pepper. Dredge in the panko and set aside. Heat 1 tablespoon of the oil in a large nonstick skillet over medium-high heat and add the shrimp. Cook until the shrimp are opaque and the bread crumbs are browned, 5 minutes; add the maple syrup, toss, and cook until the shrimp are glazed. Set aside to cool slightly. In a large bowl, toss the baby spinach with the red onion, walnuts, white wine vinegar, and remaining 1 table-spoon oil. Divide among 4 plates and top evenly with shrimp.

Yield: 4 servings (about 1¾ cups salad and 6 shrimp each)

Per serving: 304 calories; 27 g protein; 16 g carbohydrates; 2 g fiber; 7 g sugars; 14 g fat; 2 g saturated fat; 0 trans fat; 172 mg cholesterol; 361 mg sodium; 124 mg calcium; 1.3 g omega-3 fats; 4,520 IU vitamin A; 16 mg vitamin C; 3 mg vitamin E; 4.5 mg iron; 2.2 mg zinc

SWEET POTATO HASH

1 large sweet potato (12–14 ounces), cut into ½-inch dice (3 cups)
1 medium red onion, cut into large chunks (1 cup)
½ red bell pepper, cut into 1-inch pieces (¾ cup)
2 garlic cloves, sliced
1½ tablespoons extra virgin olive oil
1 teaspoon kosher salt
½ teaspoon hot red pepper flakes

Preheat the oven to 425°F. Place an empty baking sheet in the oven to heat for 5 minutes. Toss all the ingredients together in a bowl until well coated; remove the tray from the oven and spread the sweet potato mixture in a single layer. Return to the oven and cook until the potatoes are tender, 30 minutes.

Yield: 4 servings (about ¾ cup each)

Per serving: 127 calories; 2 g protein; 18 g carbohydrates; 3 g fiber; 7 g sugars; 5.5 g fat; 0.8 g saturated fat; 0 trans fat; 0 cholesterol; 505 mg sodium; 33 mg calcium; 0.1 g omega-3 fats; 13,150 IU vitamin A; 48 mg vitamin C; 2 mg vitamin E; 1 mg iron; 0.3 mg zinc

WALNUT-CRUSTED SALMON

4 6-ounce wild salmon fillets
½ teaspoon kosher salt
½ teaspoon freshly ground black pepper
½ cup walnuts, chopped very fine
2 teaspoons thyme leaves, chopped
2 teaspoons extra virgin olive oil

Preheat the oven to 425°F and line a baking sheet with aluminum foil. Place the salmon skin side down on the foil and season with the salt and pepper. Combine the walnuts and thyme and pat evenly on the salmon fillets. Drizzle with olive oil and roast until just cooked through, 7–9 minutes.

Yield: 4 servings (1 salmon filet each)

Per serving: 393 calories; 41 g protein; 2.3 g carbohydrates; 1.1 g fiber; 0.4 g sugars; 24 g fat; 3 g saturated fat; 0 trans fat; 107 mg cholesterol; 326 mg sodium; 40 mg calcium; 5 g omega-3 fats; 89 IU vitamin A; 1 mg vitamin C; 2.3 mg vitamin E; 2 mg iron; 2 mg zinc

WHITE WINE–POACHED SALMON WITH BALSAMIC ROASTED ASPARAGUS

24 ounces asparagus, trimmed
1 teaspoon extra virgin olive oil
½ teaspoon kosher salt
½ teaspoon freshly ground black pepper
1 cup thinly sliced sweet onion
½ cup dry white wine
½ cup water
1 lemon, sliced
4 sprigs fresh thyme
4 6-ounce skinless wild salmon fillets
2 teaspoons balsamic vinegar

Preheat the oven to 425°F. Place the asparagus in the center of a large piece of aluminum foil. Drizzle with olive oil, half of the salt and pepper, and ¼ cup of the sliced onion. Wrap tightly and set aside. In a shallow pan, combine the wine, water, sliced lemon, thyme, and remaining sliced onion. Bring to a simmer. Season the salmon with the remaining ¼ teaspoon each salt and pepper and add to the liquid. Turn off the burner and place the salmon and the asparagus bundle in the oven. Cook until the asparagus is tender and the salmon is cooked through, 10 minutes. Carefully open the asparagus foil bundle, drizzle with balsamic vinegar, and serve with the salmon fillets.

Yield: 4 servings (1 salmon fillet and 6 ounces asparagus each)

Per serving: 341 calories; 48 g protein; 3.5 g carbohydrates; 1.3 g fiber; 1.5 g sugars; 14 g fat; 2.9 g saturated fat; 0 trans fat; 97 mg cholesterol; 340 mg sodium; 95 mg calcium; 2.7 g omega-3 fats; 747 IU vitamin A; 6.4 mg vitamin C; 2.4 mg vitamin E; 2 mg iron; 1.2 mg zinc

The Beauty Diet Snacks

BLACK AND BLUE YOGURT PARFAIT

2 cups nonfat plain yogurt
1 teaspoon vanilla extract
1 cup blackberries
1 cup blueberries
¼ cup toasted walnuts, chopped

Combine the yogurt and vanilla until blended. To assemble the parfaits, place ¼ cup blackberries in the bottom of a parfait glass. Top with ¼ cup yogurt, ¼ cup blueberries, and another ¼ cup yogurt; top with 1 tablespoon walnuts. Repeat with the remaining 3 parfait glasses.

Yield: 4 servings (1 parfait each)

Per serving: 138 calories; 7 g protein; 19 g carbohydrates; 3 g fiber; 12 g sugars; 5 g fat; 0.5 g saturated fat; 0 trans fat; 2.5 mg cholesterol; 68 mg sodium; 170 mg calcium; 0.7 g omega-3 fats; 598 IU vitamin A; 17 mg vitamin C; 3 mg vitamin E; 0.5 mg iron; 0.5 mg zinc

BLACKBERRY YOGURT

1 cup low-fat plain yogurt
⅓ cup blackberries
1 tablespoon wheat germ

Mix the yogurt with the blackberries in a small bowl. Sprinkle with wheat germ.

Yield: 1 serving

Per serving: 202 calories; 16 g protein; 25 g carbohydrates; 3.5 g fiber; 20 g sugars; 4.8 g fat; 2.6 g saturated fat; 0 trans fat; 15 mg cholesterol; 172 mg sodium; 465 mg calcium; 0.13 g omega-3 fats; 234 IU vitamin A; 12 mg vitamin C; 2 mg vitamin E; 1.1 mg iron; 3.6 mg zinc

BLUEBERRY GINGER SMOOTHIE

1 cup blueberries
¼ cup fresh lemon juice
2 cups low-fat plain yogurt
¼ cup honey
2 teaspoons finely chopped fresh ginger

Combine all ingredients in a blender and puree until smooth. Chill or serve over ice.

Yield: 4 servings (7 ounces each)

Per serving: 167 calories; 7 g protein; 33 g carbohydrates; 1 g fiber; 30 g sugars; 2 g fat; 1 g saturated fat; 0 trans fat; 7 mg cholesterol; 87 mg sodium; 229 mg calcium; 0.04 g omega-3 fats; 85 IU vitamin A; 12 mg vitamin C; 0.3 mg vitamin E; 0.3 mg iron; 1.2 mg zinc

BLUEBERRY YOGURT PANNA COTTA

1 tablespoon gelatin
¼ cup water
2 cups buttermilk
2 cups blueberries
½ teaspoon grated orange zest
1 cup fat-free Greek yogurt
¼ cup sugar

In a small bowl, sprinkle the gelatin over 2 tablespoons of the water; set aside. Combine the buttermilk, blueberries, orange zest, and yogurt in a blender and blend until smooth. Add the rest of the water, the sugar, and the reserved gelatin to a small saucepan over medium heat and stir until well dissolved. With the blender running, add the sugar-gelatin mixture and blend until incorporated. Pour through a strainer (to remove blueberry skins and any small lumps of gelatin) into 4 serving glasses and chill until firm, about 4 hours.

Yield: 4 servings (1 generous cup each)

Per serving: 161 calories; 12 g protein; 28 g carbohydrates; 2 g fiber; 25 g sugars; 1 g fat; 0.7 g saturated fat; 0 trans fat; 8 mg cholesterol; 152 mg sodium; 193 mg calcium; 0.1 g omega-3 fats; 73 IU vitamin A; 9 mg vitamin C; 0.5 mg vitamin E; 0.4 mg iron; 1.5 mg zinc

CHERRY WALNUT GRANOLA WITH YOGURT

¾ cup old-fashioned rolled oats
2 tablespoons wheat germ
¼ cup chopped walnuts
2 tablespoons sweetened flaked coconut
1 tablespoon honey
½ teaspoon vanilla extract
1 teaspoon vegetable oil
1 tablespoon water
¼ cup dried cherries
1 quart low-fat plain yogurt

Preheat the oven to 350°F and line a baking sheet with aluminum foil. In a small bowl, mix the oats, wheat germ, walnuts, and coconut. In a separate bowl, mix together the honey, vanilla, oil, and water and stir into the dry ingredients. Spread on the prepared baking sheet in a single layer and bake for 15 minutes, stirring halfway through the cooking time, until dry and toasted. Remove from the oven, stir in the dried cherries, and let cool. Stir into the yogurt.

Yield: 4 servings (1 cup yogurt and ⅓ cup granola each)

Per serving: 336 calories; 17 g protein; 42 g carbohydrates; 5 g fiber; 25 g sugars; 12 g fat; 3.8 g saturated fat; 0 trans fat; 15 mg cholesterol; 173 mg sodium; 469 mg calcium; 1 g omega-3 fats; 414 IU vitamin A; 2.3 mg vitamin C; 1 mg vitamin E; 2 mg iron; 3.5 mg zinc

CHOCOLATE ORANGE HOT CHOCOLATE

1 quart low-fat plain milk
2 ounces dark chocolate (60 percent cacao)
1 tablespoon unsweetened cocoa powder
½ teaspoon grated orange zest

Bring the milk, chocolate, and cocoa powder to a simmer, whisking until combined. Turn off the heat and whisk in the orange zest.

Yield: 4 servings (about 1 cup each)

Per serving: 178 calories; 10 g protein; 20 g carbohydrates; 2 g fiber; 17 g sugars; 7.5 g fat; 4.7 g saturated fat; 0 trans fat; 13 mg cholesterol; 108 mg sodium; 293 mg calcium; 0.01 g omega-3 fats; 479 IU vitamin A; 0.3 mg vitamin C; 0.03 mg vitamin E; 1 mg iron; 1 mg zinc

CRANBERRY ORANGE GRANITA WITH DARK CHOCOLATE SHAVINGS

½ cup sugar
½ cup water
4 1-inch strips orange zest
Juice of 2 medium (6-ounce each) oranges (about ⅔ cup)
3 cups cranberry juice
1 ounce dark chocolate (60 percent cacao), grated

In a small saucepan, combine the sugar, water, and orange zest. Bring to a simmer, stirring, until the sugar is dissolved. Chill until cold. Remove the orange zest and add the remaining ingredients. Freeze until firm, about 6 hours or overnight. Scrape with a fork to form large flakes. Garnish with grated chocolate.

Yield: 4 servings (1 generous cup each)

Per serving: 220 calories; 1 g protein; 50 g carbohydrates; 0.5 g fiber; 46 g sugars; 3 g fat; 1.8 g saturated fat; 0 trans fat; 0 cholesterol; 8 mg sodium; 10 mg calcium; 0.1 g omega-3 fats; 98 IU vitamin A; 101 mg vitamin C; 0.5 mg vitamin E; 0.3 mg iron; 0.1 mg zinc

CREAMY CHOCOLATE CHERRY RICE PUDDING

¼ cup basmati rice, rinsed well
2½ cups low-fat milk
¼ cup sugar
⅛ teaspoon kosher salt
¼ cup dried cherries
1 teaspoon pure vanilla extract
1 egg yolk
1 ounce dark chocolate (60 percent cacao), coarsely grated

Combine the rice, milk, sugar, salt, and cherries in a medium saucepan over medium heat. Bring to a simmer, stirring occasionally, and continue to simmer until the rice is tender but not mushy, about 15 minutes. Lightly beat the vanilla and egg yolk in a small bowl, and when the rice is tender, add about ½ cup of the hot rice mixture, whisking constantly. Add back to the saucepan, whisking until slightly thickened and just returning to a simmer; remove from the heat. Pour into 4 bowls or ramekins. Refrigerate until chilled. Serve with grated chocolate on top.

Yield: 4 servings (generous ½ cup each)

Per serving: 235 calories; 7 g protein; 40 g carbohydrates; 3 g fiber; 27 g sugars; 5 g fat; 1.4 g saturated fat; 0 trans fat; 59 mg cholesterol; 130 mg sodium; 196 mg calcium; 0.02 g omega-3 fats; 643 IU vitamin A; 0 vitamin C; 0.2 mg vitamin E; 1 mg iron; 1 mg zinc

CRUNCHY DARK CHOCOLATE–DIPPED KIWIS

2 ounces dark chocolate (60 percent cacao)
8 kiwis, peeled and thickly sliced
¼ cup chopped roasted salted almonds

Heat the chocolate in a microwave-safe dish for 30-second intervals until soft; stir until smooth. Dip the kiwis in the melted chocolate. Place on wax paper and sprinkle with almonds. Chill until the chocolate solidifies.

Yield: 4 servings (4 slices each)

Per serving: 217 calories; 5 g protein; 31 g carbohydrates; 7 g fiber; 19 g sugars; 10 g fat; 3 g saturated fat; 0 trans fat; 0 cholesterol; 35 mg sodium; 75 mg calcium; 0.1 g omega-3 fats; 132 IU vitamin A; 141 mg vitamin C; 4.5 mg vitamin E; 1.4 mg iron; 0.4 mg zinc

DARK CHOCOLATE BROWNIES

⅓ cup sugar
2 tablespoons unsweetened cocoa powder
⅛ teaspoon kosher salt
¼ cup low-fat plain yogurt
½ teaspoon instant coffee
1 teaspoon warm water
1 egg
1 ounce dark chocolate (60 percent cacao), melted and cooled
2 tablespoons flour
Nonstick cooking spray

Preheat the oven to 350° F. Combine the sugar, cocoa powder, salt, and yogurt in a medium bowl and whisk until smooth. Dissolve the instant coffee in the warm water and whisk into the yogurt mixture. Whisk in the egg and then the chocolate. Stir in the flour until just combined. Divide between 4 muffin cups, sprayed with nonstick cooking spray. Bake until the edges are set and the center is soft but not wet, 18–20 minutes. Let cool completely.

Yield: 4 servings (1 brownie each)

Per serving: 148 calories; 4 g protein; 26 g carbohydrates; 2 g fiber; 20 g sugars; 4 g fat; 2 g saturated fat; 0 trans fat; 54 mg cholesterol; 90 mg sodium; 40 mg calcium; 0.01 g omega-3 fats; 69 IU vitamin A; 0.1 mg vitamin C; 0.1 mg vitamin E; 1 mg iron; 0.5 mg zinc

DARK CHOCOLATE–COVERED STRAWBERRIES

4 ounces dark chocolate (60 percent cacao)
16 strawberries

Heat the chocolate in a microwave-safe dish for 30-second intervals until soft; stir until smooth. Dip the strawberries in the melted chocolate. Place on wax paper and chill until the chocolate solidifies.

Yield: 4 servings (4 strawberries each)

Per serving: 168 calories; 3 g protein; 20 g carbohydrates; 4.5 g fiber; 14 g sugars; 10 g fat; 6 g saturated fat; 0 trans fat; 1.5 mg cholesterol; 2 mg sodium; 13 mg calcium; 0.05 g omega-3 fats; 9 IU vitamin A; 42 mg vitamin C; 0.2 mg vitamin E; 1.4 mg iron; 0.1 mg zinc

DARK CHOCOLATE–DIPPED APPLES WITH PISTACHIOS

4 ounces dark chocolate (60 percent cacao)
4 apples, cut into 6 wedges each
¼ cup chopped pistachios

Heat the chocolate in a microwave-safe dish for 30-second intervals until soft; stir until smooth. Dip the apple slices into the melted chocolate. Place on wax paper and sprinkle with pistachios. Chill until the chocolate solidifies.

Yield: 4 servings (6 apple slices each)

Per serving: 300 calories; 4.5 g protein; 46 g carbohydrates; 9 g fiber; 33 g sugars; 13 g fat; 6 g saturated fat; 0 trans fat; 1.5 mg cholesterol; 4 mg sodium; 23 mg calcium; 0.04 g omega-3 fats; 159 IU vitamin A; 10 mg vitamin C; 0.6 mg vitamin E; 1.7 mg iron; 0.3 mg zinc

DARK CHOCOLATE–DIPPED FROZEN BANANAS

4 medium bananas
4 ounces dark chocolate (60 percent cacao)
⅛ teaspoon kosher salt
2 tablespoons finely chopped walnuts

Peel the bananas and cut in half crosswise. Place on wax paper. Melt the chocolate and salt in a microwave-safe dish in 30-second intervals until soft; stir until smooth. Dip one side of the banana in the chocolate and place, chocolate side up, on the wax paper. Repeat with the remaining halves, sprinkle with walnuts, and place in the freezer for 1 to 2 hours or until the chocolate is hard and the bananas are semifrozen.

Yield: 4 servings (2 banana halves each)

Per serving: 285 calories; 4 g protein; 36 g carbohydrates; 5 g fiber; 22 g sugars; 15 g fat; 7 g saturated fat; 0 trans fat; 0 cholesterol; 76 mg sodium; 10 mg calcium; 0.4 g omega-3 fats; 76 IU vitamin A; 10 mg vitamin C; 0.1 mg vitamin E; 0.4 mg iron; 0.3 mg zinc

DARK CHOCOLATE–DIPPED PRETZELS

2 ounces dark chocolate (60 percent cacao)
16 pretzel rods

Heat the chocolate in a microwave-safe dish for 30-second intervals until soft; stir until smooth. Roll the pretzel rods in the chocolate. Place on wax paper and chill until the chocolate solidifies.

Yield: 4 servings (4 pretzel rods each)

Per serving: 217 calories; 5 g protein; 36 g carbohydrates; 3 g fiber; 7 g sugars; 6 g fat; 3 g saturated fat; 0 trans fat; 1 mg cholesterol; 488 mg sodium; 9 mg calcium; 0 omega-3 fats; 2.5 IU vitamin A; 0 vitamin C; 0 vitamin E; 2 mg iron; 0.3 mg zinc

DARK CHOCOLATE FONDUE WITH STRAWBERRIES

2 ounces dark chocolate (60 percent cacao)
½ teaspoon vanilla extract
2 cups strawberries

In a small microwave-safe bowl, microwave the chocolate in 20-second intervals until melted. Stir until smooth and then stir in the vanilla extract. If the chocolate becomes lumpy, continue to stir and microwave for 5–10 seconds, until smooth again. Serve with strawberries.

Yield: 4 servings (½ cup strawberries and ½ ounce chocolate each)

Per serving: 106 calories; 2 g protein; 11 g carbohydrates; 2.4 g fiber; 8 g sugars; 6 g fat; 3.5 g saturated fat; 0 trans fat; 0 cholesterol; 8 mg sodium; 13 mg calcium; 0.1 g omega-3 fats; 10 IU vitamin A; 49 mg vitamin C; 0.2 mg vitamin E; 0.3 mg iron; 0.1 mg zinc

GREEN TEA FROZEN YOGURT

¾ cup fat-free evaporated milk
4 green tea bags
2 cups fat-free Greek-style yogurt
¾ cup sugar

Heat the milk in a small saucepan over medium heat until steaming but not boiling. Remove from the heat, add the tea bags, and steep for 6–8 minutes. Remove the tea bags and whisk the infused milk with the yogurt and sugar. Chill until very cold, at least 1 hour and up to 24 hours. Prepare an ice cream maker according to the manufacturer's directions and add the cold green tea yogurt mixture. Churn until thick and soft-set, place in a freezer-safe plastic storage container, and freeze until hard.

Yield: 4 servings (1 cup each)

Per serving: 250 calories; 16 g protein; 48 g carbohydrates; 0 fiber; 48 g sugars; 0.1 g fat; 0.1 g saturated fat; 0 trans fat; 8 mg cholesterol; 94 mg sodium; 230 mg calcium; 0 g omega-3 fats; 189 IU vitamin A; 0.6 mg vitamin C; 0 vitamin E; 0.4 mg iron; 2.1 mg zinc

HONEY YOGURT CUP

8 ounces low-fat plain yogurt
1 tablespoon honey
2 tablespoons wheat germ

Blend the yogurt and honey in a bowl. Sprinkle with wheat germ.

Yield: 1 serving

Per serving: 261 calories; 16 g protein; 40 g carbohydrates; 2.2 g fiber; 34 g sugars; 5 g fat; 2.5 g saturated fat; 0 trans fat; 13 mg cholesterol; 160 mg sodium; 423 mg calcium; 0.14 g omega-3 fats; 130 IU vitamin A; 3 mg vitamin C; 2.3 mg vitamin E; 1.6 mg iron; 4.4 mg zinc

KIWI AND MELON FRUIT SOUP

3 kiwis (8 ounces), peeled and roughly chopped (1½ cups)
2 cups cubed honeydew melon
2 tablespoons sugar
¼ teaspoon vanilla extract
¼ cup low-fat plain yogurt for garnish
2 tablespoons chopped fresh mint for garnish

Combine the kiwi, honeydew, sugar, and vanilla in a blender and puree until smooth. Divide among four bowls and garnish each bowl with 1 tablespoon yogurt and 1½ teaspoons chopped mint.

Yield: 4 servings (generous ½ cup each)

Per serving: 87 calories; 2 g protein; 20 g carbohydrates; 2.3 g fiber; 17 g sugars; 0.6 g fat; 0 g saturated fat; 0 trans fat; 1 mg cholesterol; 28 mg sodium; 55 mg calcium; 0.1 g omega-3 fats; 208 IU vitamin A; 61 mg vitamin C; 1 mg vitamin E; 1 mg iron; 0.3 mg zinc

KIWI MELON FRUIT SALAD WITH GINGER BLUEBERRY SYRUP

4 kiwis, peeled and diced (about 2 cups)
1 cup diced honeydew
1 cup diced cantaloupe
3 tablespoons sugar
3 tablespoons water
1 teaspoon grated fresh ginger
¼ cup blueberries
1 teaspoon finely grated lemon zest

In a large bowl, combine the kiwis, honeydew, and cantaloupe; toss well. In a small saucepan, bring the sugar, water, and ginger to a boil, stirring until the sugar is dissolved, 1 minute. Stir in the blueberries and lemon zest and continue to cook until the blueberries are softened, 2 minutes. Remove from the heat and cool. Pour over the fruit and toss well.

Yield: 4 servings (about 1 cup each)

Per serving: 117 calories; 1.5 g protein; 29 g carbohydrates; 3 g fiber; 23 g sugars; 0.5 g fat; 0 saturated fat; 0 trans fat; 0 cholesterol; 16 mg sodium; 33 mg calcium; 0.1 g omega-3 fats; 1,412 IU vitamin A; 94 mg vitamin C; 1.2 mg vitamin E; 0.4 mg iron; 0.2 mg zinc

KIWI SHAKE

2 kiwis, peeled
½ banana
6 ounces low-fat vanilla yogurt

Blend the kiwis with the banana and yogurt. Pour into a glass, over ice if desired.

Yield: 1 serving

Per serving: 298 calories; 11 g protein; 61 g carbohydrates; 6.3 g fiber; 45 g sugars; 3 g fat; 1.5 g saturated fat; 0 trans fat; 8.5 mg cholesterol; 118 mg sodium; 346 mg calcium; 0.1 g omega-3 fats; 249 IU vitamin A; 148 mg vitamin C; 2.3 mg vitamin E; 1 mg iron; 2 mg zinc

LEMON SORBET WITH FRESH BLUEBERRY SAUCE

¼ cup blueberries
1 teaspoon sugar
½ cup lemon sorbet

Blend the blueberries and sugar. Serve over the lemon sorbet.

Yield: 1 serving

Per serving: 147 calories; 0.3 g protein; 37 g carbohydrates; 1.4 g fiber; 35 g sugars; 0.1 g fat; 0 g saturated fat; 0 trans fat; 0 cholesterol; 25 mg sodium; 22 mg calcium; 0.02 g omega-3 fats; 20 IU vitamin A; 6 mg vitamin C; 0.2 mg vitamin E; 0.1 mg iron; 0.1 mg zinc

LOW-FAT DOUBLE-CHOCOLATE MILK SHAKE

2 cups vanilla frozen yogurt, such as Häagen-Dazs, slightly softened
1 cup low-fat milk
2 tablespoons unsweetened cocoa powder
1½ ounces melted dark chocolate (60 percent cacao)

Place the frozen yogurt, milk, and cocoa powder in a blender and blend until smooth and thick. With the motor running, pour in the melted chocolate and blend until well mixed.

Yield: 4 servings (about ¾ cup each)

Per serving: 286 calories; 12 g protein; 40 g carbohydrates; 2 g fiber; 28 g sugars; 9 g fat; 5 g saturated fat; 0 trans fat; 68 mg cholesterol; 83 mg sodium; 326 mg calcium; 0 omega-3 fats; 319 IU vitamin A; 0 vitamin C; 0 vitamin E; 1 mg iron; 0.4 mg zinc

MANGO KIWI BLACKBERRY SMOOTHIE

4 kiwis, peeled and chopped
1 mango, peeled, pitted, and cubed
½ cup blackberries
4 ounces silken tofu
2 cups low-fat milk
¼ cup sugar

Place all the ingredients in a blender and puree until smooth. Strain if desired. Serve chilled or over ice.

Yield: 4 servings (about 1 cup each)

Per serving: 205 calories; 7.5 g protein; 41 g carbohydrates; 4 g fiber; 34 g sugars; 2.5 g fat; 1 g saturated fat; 0 trans fat; 6 mg cholesterol; 67 mg sodium; 191 mg calcium; 0.1 g omega-3 fats; 740 IU vitamin A; 89 mg vitamin C; 2 mg vitamin E; 1 mg iron; 1 mg zinc

MAPLE YOGURT CRUNCH

3 cups nonfat plain yogurt
¼ cup maple syrup
1 cup Spiced Walnuts (see Index), coarsely chopped

Mix the yogurt and maple syrup together. Place ¾ cup yogurt in a small bowl and top with ¼ cup walnuts.

Yield: 4 servings (about 1 cup each)

Per serving: 304 calories; 12 g protein; 34 g carbohydrates; 3 g fiber; 22 g sugars; 16.5 g fat; 1.5 g saturated fat; 0 trans fat; 3.8 mg cholesterol; 256 mg sodium; 275 mg calcium; 2.3 g omega-3 fats; 755 IU vitamin A; 10 mg vitamin C; 3.3 mg vitamin E; 2 mg iron; 2 mg zinc

NUTTY BANANA SHAKE

3 large bananas (about 1¼ pounds)
2 cups skim milk
2 tablespoons creamy peanut butter
2 tablespoons toasted chopped walnuts
1 teaspoon vanilla extract

Combine all the ingredients in a blender and blend until smooth. Serve over ice if desired.

Yield: 4 servings (1 cup each)

Per serving: 210 calories; 8 g protein; 32 g carbohydrates; 3.5 g fiber; 19 g sugars; 7 g fat; 1 g saturated fat; 0 trans fat; 1.5 mg cholesterol; 103 mg sodium; 137 mg calcium; 0.4 g omega-3 fats; 316 IU vitamin A; 10 mg vitamin C; 1 mg vitamin E; 0.5 mg iron; 0.5 mg zinc

PEACH BLUEBERRY GINGER CRISP

1 pound peaches, pitted and chopped (about 3 cups)
1 cup blueberries
2 tablespoons sugar
2 tablespoons flour
1 teaspoon grated fresh ginger
½ cup crushed gingersnap cookies
1 tablespoon butter, cut into 6 small pieces

Preheat the oven to 350°F. In a large bowl, toss the peaches, blueberries, sugar, flour, and ginger until well mixed and the flour has been absorbed. Place in a small baking dish, top with the crushed cookies, and dot with the butter pieces. Lightly cover with aluminum foil and bake for 15 minutes or until the fruit is bubbling around the edges. Remove the foil and continue to cook for 5–10 minutes or until the cookies have browned and crisped lightly. Let cool for at least 30 minutes. Serve warm or at room temperature.

Yield: 4 servings (about 1 cup cobbler each)

Per serving: 163 calories; 2 g protein; 31 g carbohydrates; 3 g fiber; 20 g sugars; 4 g fat; 2 g saturated fat; 0 g trans fat; 7.5 mg cholesterol; 86 mg sodium; 17 mg calcium; 0.04 g omega-3 fats; 429 IU vitamin A; 10 mg vitamin C; 1.1 mg vitamin E; 1.2 mg iron; 0.3 mg zinc

POMEGRANATE BLUEBERRY SMOOTHIE

1 cup pomegranate juice
½ cup frozen blueberries
¼ teaspoon vanilla extract

Blend the pomegranate juice with the frozen blueberries and the vanilla extract. Serve over ice if desired.

Yield: 1 serving

Per serving: 178 calories; 1.5 g protein; 44 g carbohydrates; 2 g fiber; 41 g sugars; 0.5 g fat; 0 saturated fat; 0 trans fat; 0 cholesterol; 30 mg sodium; 40 mg calcium; 0 omega-3 fats; 50 IU vitamin A; 2 mg vitamin C; 0 vitamin E; 0.5 mg iron; 0 zinc

QUARTERED FIGS DRIZZLED WITH HONEY YOGURT SAUCE AND TOASTED ALMONDS

¼ cup sliced almonds
¼ teaspoon ground ancho chile
16 ripe figs, quartered
½ cup low-fat plain yogurt
1 tablespoon honey

Preheat the oven to 350°F and line a small baking sheet with parchment paper. Toss the almonds with the ground chile and spread in a single layer on the baking sheet. Bake until toasted and lightly browned, 6–8 minutes. Let cool. Spread the fig quarters on a large plate, mix the yogurt and honey in a small bowl, drizzle over the figs, and sprinkle with toasted almond slices.

Yield: 4 servings (4 figs, 2 tablespoons yogurt, and 1 tablespoon almonds each)

Per serving: 218 calories; 4.4 g protein; 46 g carbohydrates; 7 g fiber; 39 g sugars; 4 g fat; 0.7 g saturated fat; 0 trans fat; 1.8 mg cholesterol; 25 mg sodium; 142 mg calcium; 0.01 g omega-3 fats; 348 IU vitamin A; 4.4 mg vitamin C; 2 mg vitamin E; 1 mg iron; 1 mg zinc

QUICK MEXICAN HOT DARK CHOCOLATE

1 quart low-fat milk
2 ounces dark chocolate (60 percent cacao)
½ teaspoon ground cinnamon
1 tablespoon unsweetened cocoa powder
⅛ to ¼ teaspoon cayenne, to taste

Combine all the ingredients in a small saucepan over medium heat and cook, whisking, until the chocolate is melted and the milk is just about to simmer. Serve hot.

Yield: 4 servings (1 cup each)

Per serving: 185 calories; 9.6 g protein; 18 g carbohydrates; 1.3 g fiber; 16 g sugars; 8.6 g fat; 5 g saturated fat; 0 trans fat; 12 mg cholesterol; 115 mg sodium; 296 mg calcium; 0.01 g omega-3 fats; 526 IU vitamin A; 0.2 mg vitamin C; 0.1 mg vitamin E; 0.4 mg iron; 1.1 mg zinc

RASPBERRY ALMOND YOGURT CUP

1 cup low-fat plain yogurt
2 tablespoons seedless raspberry preserves
2 tablespoons toasted chopped almonds

Blend the yogurt and raspberry preserves in a bowl. Sprinkle with almonds.

Yield: 1 serving

Per serving: 302 calories; 15 g protein; 40 g carbohydrates; 1.4 g fiber; 34 g sugars; 10 g fat; 3 g saturated fat; 0 trans fat; 15 mg cholesterol; 172 mg sodium; 478 mg calcium; 0.03 g omega-3 fats; 126 IU vitamin A; 2 mg vitamin C; 3.2 mg vitamin E; 1 mg iron; 2.6 mg zinc

RASPBERRY LEMON YOGURT CUP

1 cup low-fat plain yogurt
½ cup fresh raspberries
½ teaspoon grated lemon zest

Mix the yogurt with the raspberries in a small bowl. Sprinkle with lemon zest.

Yield: 1 serving

Per serving: 187 calories; 14 g protein; 25 g carbohydrates; 4 g fiber; 20 g sugars; 4 g fat; 2 g saturated fat; 0 trans fat; 15 mg cholesterol; 172 mg sodium; 465 mg calcium; 0.11 g omega-3 fats; 146 IU vitamin A; 19 mg vitamin C; 1 mg vitamin E; 1 mg iron; 2.4 mg zinc

ROASTED PEACHES WITH WALNUT CRUMB FILLING

4 ripe peaches (1¼ pounds)
⅓ cup finely chopped walnuts
2 teaspoons chopped crystallized ginger
2 teaspoons light brown sugar
1½ tablespoons butter, cut into small slices

Preheat the oven to 325°F. Line a baking sheet with foil; set aside. Halve the peaches, remove the pits, and place cut side up on the baking sheet. In a small bowl, mix the walnuts, ginger, and sugar and sprinkle evenly over the peach halves. Dot with butter and roast in the oven until the peaches are softened and the walnuts are toasted, 12–15 minutes.

Yield: 4 servings (2 stuffed peach halves each)

Per serving: 163 calories; 3 g protein; 17 g carbohydrates; 2.5 g fiber; 13 g sugars; 11 g fat; 3 g saturated fat; 0 trans fat; 11 mg cholesterol; 32 mg sodium; 22 mg calcium; 1 g omega-3 fats; 565 IU vitamin A; 8 mg vitamin C; 1.1 mg vitamin E; 1 mg iron; 0.5 mg zinc

SPICED WALNUTS

1 egg white
½ teaspoon salt
¼ teaspoon ground white pepper
½ teaspoon ground cinnamon
½ teaspoon ground ginger
2 cups walnut halves

Preheat the oven to 400°F. Beat the egg white and spices with a whisk until frothy. Add the walnuts and toss to coat. Spread on a baking sheet in a single layer and cook until toasted and dried, about 10 minutes. Let cool on the baking sheet; the nuts will crisp as they cool. Once cooled, the nuts can be stored in a plastic storage bag or container for up to 2 weeks.

Yield: 8 servings (¼ cup each)

Per serving: 177 calories; 5 g protein; 6 g carbohydrates; 3 g fiber; 0.7 g sugars; 16 g fat; 1.5 g saturated fat; 0 trans fat; 0 cholesterol; 153 mg sodium; 36 mg calcium; 2.3 g omega-3 fats; 5.4 IU vitamin A; 1.1 mg vitamin C; 0.3 mg vitamin E; 1.3 mg iron; 1 mg zinc

SWEET AND SPICY YOGURT

1 cup low-fat plain yogurt
1 tablespoon maple syrup
⅛ teaspoon chipotle powder
2 tablespoons toasted chopped almonds

Combine all the ingredients in a small bowl. Stir until well blended.

Yield: 1 serving

Per serving: 276 calories; 15 g protein; 33 g carbohydrates; 1.5 g fiber; 30 g sugars; 10 g fat; 2.9 g saturated fat; 0 trans fat; 15 mg cholesterol; 177 mg sodium; 492 mg calcium; 0.03 g omega-3 fats; 222 IU vitamin A; 2.2 mg vitamin C; 3.2 mg vitamin E; 1 mg iron; 3.4 mg zinc

TOMATO, MOZZARELLA, AND BASIL STACK

½ medium tomato, sliced
2 ounces sliced part-skim mozzarella
1 teaspoon balsamic vinegar
¼ cup fresh basil leaves

Layer the tomato slices with the mozzarella. Drizzle with balsamic vinegar and sprinkle with basil leaves.

Yield: 1 serving

Per serving: 180 calories; 15 g protein; 6 g carbohydrates; 1.3 g fiber; 3 g sugars; 12 g fat; 7 g saturated fat; 0 trans fat; 30 mg cholesterol; 425 mg sodium; 425 mg calcium; 0.04 g omega-3 fats; 1,580 IU vitamin A; 11.4 mg vitamin C; 0.4 mg vitamin E; 1 mg iron; 0.2 mg zinc

TROPICAL KIWI FRUIT SALAD WITH VANILLA LIME SYRUP

3 kiwis, peeled and diced (1½ cups)
1 ripe mango, peeled and diced (1½ cups)
½ cored pineapple, diced (about 1½ cups)
2 tablespoons water
2 tablespoons sugar
½ vanilla bean
½ teaspoon grated lime zest
¼ cup sweetened flaked coconut

In a medium bowl, combine the kiwis, mango, and pineapple. Set aside. Put the water and sugar into a small saucepan, then split the vanilla bean lengthwise, scrape the seeds into the pan, and add the pod. Bring to a simmer and cook until the sugar is dissolved, about 1 minute. Let cool, remove the vanilla pod, stir in the lime zest, and pour over the fruit. Toss well and chill for 1–2 hours to allow the flavors to mingle. Add the coconut before serving.

Yield: 4 servings (1 cup each)

Per serving: 149 calories; 1.4 g protein; 34 g carbohydrates; 4 g fiber; 26 g sugars; 2 g fat; 1 g saturated fat; 0 trans fat; 0 cholesterol; 5 mg sodium; 34 mg calcium; 0.1 g omega-3 fats; 556 IU vitamin A; 91 mg vitamin C; 1.6 mg vitamin E; 0.5 mg iron; 0.3 mg zinc

VANILLA ORANGE "CREAMSICLE" SMOOTHIE

2½ cups low-fat plain yogurt
1 teaspoon vanilla extract
1½ cups fresh orange juice
¼ cup sugar

Combine all the ingredients in a blender and puree until smooth. Serve well chilled.

Yield: 4 servings (1 cup each)

Per serving: 190 calories; 9 g protein; 33 g carbohydrates; 0.2 g fiber; 31 g sugars; 2.5 g fat; 1.5 g saturated fat; 0 trans fat; 9 mg cholesterol; 108 mg sodium; 291 mg calcium; 0.03 g omega-3 fats; 264 IU vitamin A; 48 mg vitamin C; 0.1 mg vitamin E; 0.3 mg iron; 1.4 mg zinc

WHITE BEAN "HUMMUS"

1 15.5-ounce can cannellini beans, drained and rinsed
1 teaspoon extra virgin olive oil
¼ cup nonfat plain yogurt
1 tablespoon fresh lemon juice
¼ teaspoon grated lemon zest
2 tablespoons chopped fresh chives
¼ teaspoon kosher salt
¼ teaspoon freshly ground black pepper

Combine all the ingredients in a food processor or blender. Puree until smooth.

Yield: 4 servings (⅓ cup each)

Per serving: 113 calories; 7 g protein; 18 g carbohydrates; 5 g fiber; 3 g sugars; 2 g fat; 0 saturated fat; 0 trans fat; 0 cholesterol; 327 mg sodium; 70 mg calcium; 0.12 g omega-3 fats; 68 IU vitamin A; 4.3 mg vitamin C; 0.2 mg vitamin E; 1.4 mg iron; 0.7 mg zinc

Index